The QCS Pool Activity Level (PAL) Instrument for Occupational Profiling

by the same author

From Dementia to Rementia
Jackie Pool
ISBN 978 1 83997 315 4
eISBN 978 1 83997 316 1

of related interest

About University of Bradford Dementia Good Practice Guides
Under the editorship of Professor Murna Downs, this series constitutes
a set of accessible, jargon-free, evidence-based good practice guides for
all those involved in the care of people with dementia and their families.
The series draws together a range of evidence, including the experience
of people with dementia and their families, practice wisdom, and
research and scholarship to promote quality of life and quality of care.

End of Life Care for People with Dementia
A Person-Centred Approach
Laura Middleton-Green, Jane Chatterjee, Sarah Russell and Murna Downs
ISBN 978 1 84905 047 0
eISBN 978 0 85700 512 0

Developing Excellent Care for People Living with Dementia in Care Homes
Caroline Baker
ISBN 978 1 84905 467 6
eISBN 978 1 78450 053 5

Leadership for Person-Centred Dementia Care
Buz Loveday
ISBN 978 1 84905 229 0
eISBN 978 0 85700 691 2

Playfulness and Dementia
A Practice Guide
John Killick
ISBN 978 1 84905 223 8
eISBN 978 0 85700 462 8

The QCS Pool Activity Level (PAL) Instrument *for* Occupational Profiling

A Practical Resource for Carers of People with Cognitive Impairment

Fifth Edition

Jackie Pool

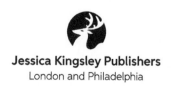

Jessica Kingsley Publishers
London and Philadelphia

Previous editions published in 1999, 2002, 2008 and 2012 by Jessica Kingsley Publishers

This fifth edition first published in Great Britain in 2023 by Jessica Kingsley Publishers
An imprint of Hodder & Stoughton Ltd
An Hachette UK Company

1

A CIP catalogue record for this title is available from the British Library and the Library of Congress

ISBN 978 1 83997 502 8
eISBN 978 1 83997 503 5

Printed and bound in Great Britain by CPI Group (UK) Ltd, Croydon, CR0 4YY

Jessica Kingsley Publishers' policy is to use papers that are natural, renewable and recyclable products and made from wood grown in sustainable forests. The logging and manufacturing processes are expected to conform to the environmental regulations of the country of origin.

Jessica Kingsley Publishers
Carmelite House
50 Victoria Embankment
London EC4Y 0DZ

www.jkp.com

CONTENTS

ABOUT THE AUTHOR AND CONTRIBUTORS

THE AUTHOR

Jackie Pool DipCOT

Jackie is an occupational therapist specializing in dementia care. She qualified in 1988 and, following her work as a clinical practitioner in the NHS and local authority, formed her own organization, Jackie Pool Associates Ltd, which specialized in resources for leadership and workforce development in dementia care. In 2021, QCS Quality Compliance Systems acquired the PAL Instrument and Jackie joined them as Dementia Care Champion. Jackie was a member of the Department of Health External Reference Group for the National Dementia Strategy. She was commissioned by Skills for Care to develop the national qualifications and credit framework dementia qualification structure and has published several works on the care of older people with dementia, including books, journal articles, training manuals and chapters in textbooks. Jackie is also a regular speaker at national and international conferences on the subject of dementia care.

THE CONTRIBUTORS

Sarah Mould DipCOT

Sarah is Specialist Practitioner for Dementia/Delirium at University Hospitals Southampton NHS Foundation Trust. Prior to that, Sarah was Co-Director of the Dementia Training Company, which specializes in the delivery of dementia training and consultation services both in the UK and internationally. Sarah worked with Jackie Pool as Director of Training with Jackie Pool Associates Ltd for many years and, as an occupational therapist by profession, she has been delighted to be a contributing author for the PAL Instrument. Sarah is a committed and passionate advocate for person-centred and rights-based approaches in the care and support of people with dementia and their caregivers.

Jennifer Wenborn MSc DipCOT

Jennifer has worked as an occupational therapist for over 30 years, predominantly with older people. She has wide experience in hospital and community settings, providing physical and mental health services, as a clinician and manager, and has also worked as an independent practitioner. She is currently a clinical research fellow in occupational therapy at University College London. The PAL study was the first phase in her PhD research, a randomized controlled trial entitled 'Does occupational therapy intervention for people with dementia in a care home setting improve quality of life?' Jennifer has written extensively about activity provision within care homes, including co-authoring *The Successful Activity Co-ordinator* in 2005, published by Age Concern.

Professor David Challis PhD

Professor of Community Care Research and Director of the Personal Social Services Research Unit at the University of Manchester, David has been responsible for a series of evaluations of the effectiveness and efficiency of intensive care management for older people, which were influential in the development of community care services in the UK. He has also acted as an advisor on care management to a number of governments and service providers in the USA, Canada, Australia and Japan. His current areas of activity include a range of studies on assessment of older people and patterns of service provision. He has authored 19 books and written over 150 articles and chapters in books.

Professor Martin Orrell PhD FRCPsych

Martin is Professor of Ageing and Mental Health at University College London (UCL) and North East London Mental Health Trust (NELMHT). He trained at the Maudsley Hospital and the Institute of Psychiatry before being appointed at UCL in 1991. At NELMHT, he works as an honorary consultant old age psychiatrist and is Associate Medical Director for Mental Health Services for Older People, and Director of Research and Development. In recent years, he has also worked as a specialist advisor to the Health Advisory Service and clinical advisor to the Audit Commission for the Forget Me Not national study on mental health services for older people. His research interests include needs assessment, health services evaluation and psychosocial interventions for dementia and he has published over 100 academic papers. He is Editor of the journal *Aging and Mental Health*, course director for the MSc in Ageing and Mental Health at UCL and Director of the London Centre for Dementia Care.

Professor Lesley Collier PhD MSc DipCOT

Lesley is Head of Allied Health at the faculty of Health and Well-being at the University of Winchester. She has worked as an occupational therapist with a focus on neurology and care of older people for 30 years. More recently, she has worked at the University of Southampton as Programme Lead for Occupational Therapy, and Brunel University London as Divisional Lead for Occupational Therapy and Nursing. Lesley's research focuses on the use of sensory approaches to improve functional performance in older people with dementia. She has published extensively in this field and has led a number of international workshops supporting others in implementing this approach.

PREFACE

This fifth edition of this guidebook provides readers with updates on the ownership of the Pool Activity Level (PAL) Instrument, which is now run by QCS Quality Compliance Systems. The QCS PAL Instrument in this new edition contains the same reliable and valid PAL Checklist and Profiles, and new to this edition is also the QCS PAL Engagement Measure. All are free to photocopy from this book.

There is also now a digital version of QCS PAL Instrument which is free to access at www.qcs.co.uk/digital-pool-activity-level-pal-instrument. Completion of this digital PAL checklist automatically calculates the abilities of the individual and creates a comprehensive PAL guide accordingly. The PAL Guide provides details of how to support the person at any of the four PAL levels of ability, across five everyday activities: dining, washing, dressing, interacting and engaging in leisure activities.

In addition, QCS has developed a wealth of supporting resources, including webinars for delivering training on using the PAL Instrument and Purposeful Practice Guides to develop care practice skills and competency. These can be subscribed to at the QCS Dementia Centre: www.qcs.co.uk/dementia-centre.

In this fifth edition book, in addition to the Life History, Checklist and Profiles, which help to match abilities with activities, there is an update to the Individual Activity Plans to support the delivery of personal care that facilitates a person's engagement in each of the three activities of getting dressed, bathing/washing and dining.

There is also the new addition of the PAL Engagement Measure. This final part of the PAL Instrument battery of tools has been developed and validated with the support of the Occupational Therapy Department at the University of Brunel, and with input from Professor Lesley Collier, Programme Lead at the University of Winchester, Faculty of Health and Well-being.

The Engagement Measure enables organizations and individuals to holistically measure the ability of the person using their service, with a traffic light and scoring system to review and evidence cognitive, physical, emotional and social ability over time during engagement in a chosen activity.

The Pool Activity Level (PAL) Instrument was first published in 1999 as a part of the Good Practice Guide series from the University of Bradford Dementia Group. In 2002, following feedback information from a range of users, a new version of the PAL Checklist and Action Plans was developed and a second edition of the PAL book was published.

In 2005, a research study into the effectiveness of the PAL Checklist was undertaken by University College London and the reliability and validity of the PAL Instrument was proved. The fact that the PAL Checklist was now standardized became of interest to strategic level providers and commissioners of health and social care services as a standardized assessment and outcome measure.

In the national clinical practice guideline for dementia (National Institute for Clinical

Excellence 2006), the PAL Instrument is recommended for the activity of daily living skills training and for activity planning.

This latest edition of the QCS PAL guidebook brings PAL users up to date with additional information to support them in their use of the PAL Instrument, including access to the new digital version of the PAL, powered by QCS Quality Compliance Systems, and the PAL Engagement Measure.

This book is designed to enable carers at home and in formal care settings to use the PAL Instrument to engage people with cognitive impairment in meaningful occupation. It supports a move from viewing everyday personal chores such as dining, dressing and having a wash as 'tasks' to skilling individuals to enable others to engage fully and so experience these as personal 'activities'.

People with cognitive impairments may also have difficulty engaging in activities, particularly if the activity is too demanding or not presented to the person in an understandable way. Care staff trying to provide leisure activity programmes can be at a loss to know how to offer the activity to maximize success, or how to find equipment locally or nationally. To assist carers in facilitating leisure activities, Part 2 of this guide includes ideas for four activity packs. A selection of possible activities is described, with updated sources for obtaining more information and guidance for carrying them out with individuals who have different levels of ability, as revealed by the completion of the PAL Instrument Checklist.

The PAL Instrument has become the framework for care in settings across the world for clients with cognitive impairments caused by conditions related to dementia, strokes and learning disabilities. It has been translated into many languages and continues to grow as the tool of choice for supporting people to live well with their cognitive disability.

REFERENCE

National Institute for Clinical Excellence (NICE) (2006) *Dementia: Supporting People with Dementia and their Carers in Health and Social Care*. National Clinical Practice Guideline number 42. London: NICE.

Part 1

QCS POOL ACTIVITY LEVEL (PAL) INSTRUMENT

Chapter 1

QCS POOL ACTIVITY LEVEL (PAL) INSTRUMENT

DIRECTIONS

This copy of the QCS PAL Instrument, including the Checklist, Profile, Individual Action Plan and Engagement Measure, may be photocopied for your manual use with the people for whom you care.

The digital version of the QCS PAL Instrument, which can be downloaded at www.qcs.co.uk/digital-pool-activity-level-pal-instrument, will automatically calculate the abilities of the individual from the completed Checklist to create the PAL Guide: an expanded version of the Profile, that applies understanding of the level of ability of the individual to a range of personal care and leisure activities.

COMPLETING THE PAL LIFE HISTORY PROFILE

The aim is to gather and record information that will improve the opportunities for the person with cognitive impairment to engage in meaningful activity. Completion of the Life History Profile will depend on what sections are relevant, what information is available and what the person wishes to be recorded. The headings in each section are intended as a guide. This is likely to be an ongoing process rather than a once-only task and can become a meaningful activity with the person in itself.

COMPLETING THE PAL CHECKLIST

Consider how the person with cognitive impairment generally functions when carrying out the activities described in the Checklist. If you are unsure, observe the person in the situations over a period of two weeks. If the person lives in a group setting, such as a care home, you might need to ask other caregivers for their observations too.

For each activity, the statements refer to a different level of ability. Thinking of the last two weeks, tick the statement that represents the person's ability in each activity. There should be one tick for each activity. If in doubt about which statement to tick, choose the level of ability that represents their average performance over the last two weeks. Make sure you tick only one statement for each of the activities.

When possible, complete the PAL Checklist as a team assessment so that knowledge of the person's ability is included from a range of staff.

You can decide when to complete repeat assessments using the PAL Checklist, but ideally you should do so when you notice any significant changes in the person's abilities and also as part of any care plan reviews.

INTERPRETING THE CHECKLIST

People do not fit neatly into boxes, and the PAL Instrument is designed to describe people in simple terms so that it is widely applicable. Add up the number of ticks for each activity level and enter the number in the total box at the end of the Checklist. You should find that there is a majority of ticks in one of the levels. This indicates which PAL Activity Profile to select. If the number of ticks is almost evenly divided between two activity levels, assume that the person is currently functioning at the lower level of ability for the purpose of selecting the Activity Profile, but ensure that the person has an opportunity to move into the higher level of ability.

This is a general description of the environment in which the person is likely to best engage in personal care, social and leisure activities. The box at the end of the PAL Activity Profile should be completed by referring to the information gathered and recorded in the Life History Profile. This is how the general nature of the PAL Activity Profile becomes individualized.

The PAL Activity Profiles for multisensory environments have been created to support sensory activities for individuals at each activity level, as identified by the PAL Checklist. Detailed information about multisensory activities can be found in Chapter 10.

COMPLETING THE INDIVIDUAL ACTION PLAN

Note the overall level of ability of the person and select the Individual Action Plan to support your personal care in order to facilitate the person's engagement in each of the three activities of getting dressed, bathing/washing and dining. Enter additional information about the person's preferences and routines in the spaces provided to make the Action Plan even more individualized. Use the additional notes to record any specific information that you have about the best way of supporting the person in these activities of daily living.

COMPLETING THE DIGITAL PAL GUIDE

If you are using the digital version of the PAL Instrument, your completion of the PAL Checklist will have automatically calculated the level of ability and will produce the PAL Guide for you. This Guide is a combined version of the PAL Profile and the Individual Action Plan from this book and provides information about how to support the person at their identified level of ability in a range of five activities: getting dressed; dining; bathing/showering; interacting; and leisure activities. As the PAL Guide is saved digitally as a writable document, you can further personalize it with information about the individual's preferences, routines and wishes.

COMPLETING THE ENGAGEMENT MEASURE

Use one Engagement Measure sheet for each personal care or leisure activity that you wish to record for the person. There are five columns for you to record five separate events of the activity. You can decide the frequency of the recording: for example, it could be weekly, fortnightly or monthly. The aim is to have a record of the maintenance or change in ability over time. You can record the abilities in each cell of the column with a numerical score as shown in the key: zero for not observed during the activity; one point for observed but not consistently; and two points for engaged consistently in keeping with the activity. You can also colour code your entries on the sheet with red for zero, yellow for one and green for two points. This will provide you with a graphic representation of the person's engagement over the five times of recording. Use this record to monitor the impact of your support on the person.

If you notice that there has been a significant change in the cognitive abilities or the social interaction of the person, you should complete another PAL Checklist as the person may need supporting in a different way. If you notice that there has been a significant change in physical abilities or emotional well-being, you may need to refer the person for a medical assessment.

QCS POOL ACTIVITY LEVEL (PAL) PERSONAL HISTORY PROFILE

The purpose of a Personal History Profile is to enable carers to recognize the person as a unique individual and not see only the person's disability. By finding out about all that the person has experienced, it is possible to have a better understanding of their current behaviour. It also gives care workers, who do not know the person very well, topics of conversation that will have meaning for the person.

Putting together the Profile should be an enjoyable project that the person with dementia, their relatives and care workers can all join in with, encouraging life review and reminiscence. The information gained from the Personal History Profile informs the PAL Activity Profile by guiding activity selection.

The questions in the Profile are very general, designed to cater for all people regardless of age or sex. Some questions may be irrelevant, so just ignore these!

If you can include any photographs to add to this Profile, write on the reverse:

- the person's name
- who is in the photo
- where and when it was taken.

If you are worried about the photographs getting lost or damaged, you could get them photocopied.

QCS POOL ACTIVITY LEVEL (PAL)
PERSONAL HISTORY PROFILE

What is your name?

. . . .

When were you born?

. . . .

CHILDHOOD
Where were you born?

. . . .

What are your family members' names?

. . . .

. . . .

What were your family members' occupations?

. . . .

. . . .

Where did you live?

. . . .

Which schools did you attend?

. . . .

. . . .

What was your favourite subject?

. . . .

Did you have any family pets? What were their names?

. . . .

. . . .

ADOLESCENCE
When did you leave school?

. . . .

Where did you work?

. . . .

What did you do at work?

· ·

· ·

Did you have any special training?

· ·

· ·

· ·

What special memories do you have of work days?

· ·

· ·

· ·

ADULTHOOD

Do/did you have a partner? What is your partner's name and occupation?

· ·

Where and when did you meet?

· ·

· ·

Where and when did you marry?

· ·

Where did you go on honeymoon?

· ·

Where did you live?

· ·

Do you have any children? What are their names?

· ·

Do you have any grandchildren? What are their names?

· ·

Did you have any special friends? What are their names?

· ·

When and where did you meet?

. . . .

Are they still in touch?

. . . .

Did you have any pets? What were their names?

. . . .

RETIREMENT
When did you retire?

. . . .

What were you looking forward to most?

. . . .

. . . .

What were your hobbies and interests?

. . . .

. . . .

What were the biggest changes for you?

. . . .

. . . .

LIKES AND DISLIKES
What do you enjoy doing now?

. . . .

. . . .

What do you like to read?

. . . .

. . . .

What is your favourite colour?

. . . .

What kind of music do you like?

. . . .

What are your favourite foods and drinks?

. . . .

Is there anything that you definitely do not like to do?

. . . .

. . . .

How do you like to do things? Do you have any special routines to your day?

. . . .

. . . .

What time do you like to get up in the morning? And go to bed at night?

. . . .

. . . .

Do you want people to help you with anything?

. . . .

. . . .

. . . .

Do you want people to leave you to do anything on your own?

. . . .

. . . .

. . . .

How do you like people to address you?

. . . .

What are you good at?

. . . .

. . . .

. . . .

Is there anything else you would like to tell us about you?

. . . .

. . . .

. . . .

QCS POOL ACTIVITY LEVEL (PAL) CHECKLIST

Name: . . . .

Date: . . . .

Completed by: . . . .

> Activity Level indicated: . . . .

Ensure you are familiar with the instructions before completion.

Completing the Checklist	Key
• Thinking of the last two weeks, tick the statement that represents the person's ability in each section.	P = Planned level of ability
• If in doubt about which statement to tick, choose the level of ability that represents their average performance over the last two weeks.	E = Exploratory level of ability S = Sensory level of ability
• There should only be ONE TICK for each section.	R = Reflex level of ability
• You must tick one statement for each section.	
• Total the ticks at the bottom of each column over page.	

1. Bathing/Washing	P	E	S	R
• Can bathe/wash independently, sometimes with a little help to start				
• Needs soap put on flannel and one-step-at-a-time directions to wash				
• Mainly relies on others but will wipe own face and hands if encouraged				
• Totally dependent and needs full assistance to wash or bathe				
2. Getting dressed	P	E	S	R
• Plans what to wear, selects own clothing from the cupboards; dresses in correct order				
• Needs help to plan what to wear but recognizes items and how to wear them; needs help with order of dressing				
• Needs help to plan and with order of dressing, but can carry out small activities if someone directs each step				
• Totally dependent on someone to plan, sequence and complete dressing; may move limbs to assist				
3. Eating	P	E	S	R
• Eats independently and using the correct cutlery				
• Eats using a spoon and/or needs food to be cut up into small pieces				
• Only uses fingers to eat food				
• Relies on others to be fed				

4. Contact with others	P	E	S	R
• Initiates social contact and responds to the needs of others				
• Aware of others and will seek interaction, but may be more concerned with own needs				
• Aware of others but waits for others to make the first social contact				
• May not show an awareness of the presence of others unless in direct physical contact				

5. Groupwork skills	P	E	S	R
• Engages with others in a group activity, can take turns with the activity/tools				
• Occasionally engages with others in a group, moving in and out of the group at a whim				
• Aware of others in the group and will work alongside others, although tends to focus on own activity				
• Does not show awareness of others in the group unless close one-to-one attention is experienced				

6. Communication skills	P	E	S	R
• Is aware of appropriate interaction, can chat coherently and is able to use complex language skills				
• Body language may be inappropriate and may not always be coherent, but can use simple language skills				
• Responses to verbal interaction may be mainly through body language; comprehension is limited				
• Can only respond to direct physical contact from others through touch, eye contact or facial expression				

7. Practical activities (craft, domestic chores, gardening)	P	E	S	R
• Can plan to carry out an activity, hold the goal in mind and work through a familiar sequence; may need help solving problems				
• More interested in the making or doing than the end result, needs prompting to remember purpose, can get distracted				
• Activities need to be broken down and presented one step at a time, multisensory stimulation can help hold the attention				
• Unable to 'do' activities, but responds to the close contact of others and experiencing physical sensations				

8. Use of objects	P	E	S	R
• Plans to use and looks for objects that are not visible; may struggle if objects are not in usual/familiar places (e.g. toiletries in a bathroom cupboard)				
• Selects objects appropriately only if in view (e.g. toiletries on a shelf next to the washbasin)				
• Randomly uses objects as chances on them; may use appropriately				
• May grip objects when placed in the hand but will not attempt to use them				

9. Looking at a newspaper/magazine	P	E	S	R
• Comprehends and shows interest in the content, turns the pages and looks at headlines and pictures				
• Turns the pages randomly, only attending to items pointed out by others				
• Will hold and may feel the paper, but will not turn the pages unless directed and will not show interest in the content				
• May grip the paper if it is placed in the hand but may not be able to release the grip; or may not take hold of the paper				
NB: If the totals are evenly divided between activity levels, assume that the person is at the lower level but has the potential to move into the higher level. **Totals**				

The Activity Level identified for this person is: . . . .

Transfer this information to the front of the form.

> Now use the relevant PAL Activity Profile to assist you to plan how you will help the person with their activities.

QCS PAL ACTIVITY PROFILE

PLANNED ACTIVITY LEVEL OF ABILITY

Name: . . . .

Date:. . . . .

Likely abilities

- Can explore different ways of carrying out an activity
- Can work towards completing a task with a tangible result
- Can look in obvious places for any objects

Likely limitations

- May not be able to solve problems that arise
- May not be able to understand complex sentences
- May not search beyond the usual places for objects

Caregiver's role

- To enable the person to take control of the activity and master the steps involved
- To encourage the person to initiate social interactions
- To solve problems as they arise

Using the PAL Activity Profile to support the person

Position of objects	Ensure that objects and materials are in their usual, familiar places.
Verbal directions	Explain activity using short sentences by avoiding using connecting phrases such as 'and', 'but', 'therefore' or 'if'. Allow time for a response. Repeat the directions if the person is struggling to recall the guidance. Using gentle prompts, encourage the person to solve problems encountered.
Demonstrated directions	Show the person how to avoid possible errors. If problems cannot be solved independently then demonstrate the solution. Encourage the person then to copy.
Working with others	The person is able to make the first contact and should be encouraged and be given opportunity to initiate social contact.
Activity characteristics	There is a goal or end product, with a set process, or 'recipe', to achieve it.

✓

Suitable leisure activities

- Identify an activity of interest to the person based on knowledge of their interests, career, home life and so on, or select one of the activities suggested below as a starting point.
- Ensure the task you select is not overly complex.
- An element of competition with others is motivating.
  - Memory games, newspapers, exercise activities, art/craft, board games, computer games, conversation, cooking, gardening, DIY, word quizzes/crosswords.

Activity plan:

QCS PAL ACTIVITY PROFILE

EXPLORATORY ACTIVITY LEVEL OF ABILITY

Name: . . . .

Date: . . . .

Likely abilities

- Can carry out very familiar tasks in familiar surroundings
- Enjoys the experience of doing a task more than the end result
- Can carry out more complex tasks if they are broken down into two- to three-step stages

Likely limitations

- May not have an end result in mind when starts a task
- May not recognize when the task is completed
- Relies on cues such as diaries, newspaper, lists and labels

Caregiver's role

- To enable the person to experience the sensation of doing the activity rather than focusing on the end result
- To break the activity into manageable chunks
- To keep directions simple and understandable
- To approach and make first contact as it is rarely initiated by the person

Using the PAL Activity Profile to support the person

Position of objects	Ensure that objects and materials are in the line of vision.
Verbal directions	Explain task using short simple sentences. Avoid using connecting phrases such as 'and', 'but' or 'therefore'. Also avoid using prepositions such as 'in', 'by' or 'for'. Repeat the directions if the person is struggling to recall the guidance.
Demonstrated directions	Break the activity into two or three steps at a time.
Working with others	Others must approach the person and make the first contact.
Activity characteristics	There is no pressure to perform to a set of rules, or to achieve an end result. There is an element of creativity and spontaneity.

✓

Suitable leisure activities

- Identify an activity of interest to the person based on knowledge of their interests, career, home life and so on, or select one of the activities suggested below as a starting point.
  - Outings, newspaper discussions, exercise activities, art/craft, food tasting, board games, computer games, reminiscence objects, conversation, cooking, gardening, DIY, flower arranging.

Activity plan:

QCS PAL ACTIVITY PROFILE

SENSORY ACTIVITY LEVEL OF ABILITY

Name: . . . .

Date: . . . .

Likely abilities

- Is likely to be responding to bodily sensations
- Can be guided to carry out single-step activities
- Can carry out more complex activities if they are broken down into one step at a time

Likely limitations

- May not have any conscious plan to carry out a movement to achieve a particular end result
- May be relying on others to make social contact

Caregiver's role

- To enable the person to experience the effect of the activity on his/her senses
- To break the activity into one step at a time
- To keep directions simple and understandable
- To approach and make the first contact with the person

Using the PAL Activity Profile to support the person

Position of objects	Ensure that the person becomes aware of objects and materials by making bodily contact.
Verbal directions	Limit requests to carry out actions to the naming of the action and of the object involved, e.g. 'lift your arm', 'hold the brush'.
Demonstrated directions	Demonstrate to the person the action on the object. Break the activity down into one step at a time.
Working with others	Others must approach the person and make the first contact. Use touch and the person's name to sustain the social contact.
Activity characteristics	The activity is used as an opportunity for a sensory experience. This may be multisensory. Repetitive actions are appropriate.

✓

Suitable leisure activities

- Identify an activity of interest to the person based on knowledge of their interests, career, home life and so on, or select one of the activities suggested below as a starting point.
  - Sensory box, smells, food tasting, hand massage, exercises, music and singing, dancing, sweeping, polishing, wiping tables and so on.

Activity plan:

QCS PAL ACTIVITY PROFILE

REFLEX ACTIVITY LEVEL OF ABILITY

Name: . . . .

Date:. . . . .

Likely abilities

- Can make reflex responses to direct sensory stimulation
- Direct sensory stimulation can increase awareness of self and others
- May respond to social engagement through the use of body language

Likely limitations

- May not be aware of the surrounding environment or even of his/her own body
- May have difficulty organizing the multiple sensations that are being experienced
- May become agitated in an environment that is over-stimulating

Caregiver's role

- To enable the person to be more aware of themselves
- To arouse the person to be more aware of his/her surroundings
- To engage with the person through direct sensory stimulation
- To monitor the environment and reduce multiple stimuli, loud noises and background sounds

Using the PAL Activity Profile to support the person

Position of objects	Direct stimuli to the area of body being targeted, e.g. stroke the person's arm before placing it in a sleeve, use light across the person's field of vision to encourage eye movement.
Verbal directions	Limit spoken directions to movement directions, e.g. 'lift', 'hold', 'open'. Use a warm, reassuring tone and adapt volume to establish a connection with the person.
Demonstrated directions	Guide movements by touching the relevant body part.
Working with others	Maintain eye contact, make maximum use of facial expression, gestures and body posture for a non-verbal conversation. Use social actions which can be imitated, e.g. smiling, waving, shaking hands.
Activity characteristics	The activity focuses on a single sensation: touch, smell, sound, sight, taste.

✓

Suitable leisure activities

- Identify an activity of interest to the person based on knowledge of their interests, career, home life and so on, or select one of the activities suggested below as a starting point.
  - Smells, food tasting, hand massage, music, lights, textured objects, chimes, sensory mobiles.

Activity plan:

QCS PAL ACTIVITY PROFILE FOR MULTISENSORY ENVIRONMENTS

PLANNED ACTIVITY LEVEL OF ABILITY

Name: . . . .

Date:. . . . .

Likely abilities

- Can explore different ways of engaging with a sensory activity
- Can concentrate on engaging with sensory objects and engage in communication
- Can look in obvious places for appropriate or preferred objects

Likely limitations

- May not be able to solve problems that arise while attempting to engage with sensory objects
- May not be able to understand complex sentences particularly if multisensory terms are used, e.g. bubble tube, optic fibres
- May not search beyond the usual places for multisensory objects

Caregiver's role

- To enable the person to take control of the activity and master the steps involved
- To encourage the person to initiate social interactions
- To solve problems as they arise

Using the PAL Activity Profile to support the person

Position of objects	Place the objects in the same place for each session to help orientate the person. If you are using a sensory room, orientate the person to the room on each occasion. Give them a choice of where they wish to sit. Ask the person to select preferred objects, ensuring that the selection includes stimuli for all the senses (sight, sound, touch, taste, smell and movement). Show the person different objects to help them choose. Offer no more than two or three choices at any one time.
Verbal directions	Explain the activity in short sentences and repeat directions as necessary. Avoid using connecting phrases such as 'and', 'but' or 'therefore'. Allow time for the person to respond. If the person is new to the sensory activity then demonstrate to them what is available. Demonstration will also help prevent errors in selection. Encourage the person to solve problems through gentle prompts.

Demonstrated directions and Working with others	Allow the person time to settle before focusing on the sensory aspects of the activity. If you are using a sensory room start with main room lights on and slowly dim the room. The session may last up to 30 minutes, but end the session when the person is no longer able to concentrate on the experience. The ideal session should be one-to-one but a group of up to three people may be accommodated. Allow the person time to explore and handle the objects. Focus any conversation towards what is happening, what the effect is, how it feels, the person's likes and dislikes, what it reminds them of. Encourage the person to reflect on the sensory qualities of the session with those around them. Slowly brighten the room and return the conversation to everyday discussion. Encourage the person to tidy the objects away.
Activity characteristics	There is an end goal with an enabling process. The interaction with the caregiver is an important element of this activity.

Details of multisensory activity: which pieces of equipment were selected and length of the session, any specific details regarding the caregiver's interaction with the person.

Activity plan: list other sensory activities that match a person's activity profile that can support this multisensory activity, e.g. baking, gardening.

QCS PAL ACTIVITY PROFILE FOR MULTISENSORY ENVIRONMENTS

EXPLORATORY ACTIVITY LEVEL OF ABILITY

Name: . . . .

Date: . . . .

Likely abilities

- Can carry out very familiar tasks in familiar surroundings
- Enjoys the experience of doing a task more than the end result
- Can carry out more complex tasks if they are broken down into two- to three-step stages

Likely limitations

- May not have an end result in mind when starts a task
- May not recognize when a task is completed
- Relies on cues to orientate themselves

Caregiver's role

- To enable the person to experience the sensation of doing the activity
- To break the activity down into manageable chunks
- To keep directions simple and understandable
- To approach and make first contact as it is rarely initiated by the person

Using the PAL Activity Profile to support the person

Position of objects	Lay out the selection of objects that is suitable for the person based on sensory preferences and needs, but allow for some element of choice by offering two objects at a time. Introduce the objects in a familiar surrounding such as a sitting room. Ensure the objects are in the line of vision and are easily accessible. Ensure the selection provides stimuli for all the senses (sight, sound, touch, taste, smell, movement).
Verbal directions	Explain the task in short sentences. Avoid using connecting phrases such as 'and', 'but' or 'therefore'. Also avoid using prepositions such as 'in', 'by' or 'for'. Repeat the directions if the person is struggling to recall the guidance. If the person is new to the multisensory objects then demonstrate what is available. Demonstration will also prevent errors in selection.

Demonstrated directions and Working with others	Allow the person time to settle before focusing on the sensory aspects of the session. Start with main room lights on and slowly dim the room. The session may last for up to 20 minutes, but end the session if the person is no longer able to concentrate on the task or if they fall asleep (this approach is designed to stimulate rather than relax).
	The ideal session should be one-to-one but a group of two may be accommodated.
	Break each activity down into two to three steps at a time and limit the stimulus to no more than three sensory objects operating at any one time. If the person appears distracted by the number of items operating, limit them to two.
	Allow the person to explore and handle the objects. Do not enforce any instructions on how to use or handle the objects unless the person is placing themselves in danger. Encourage the person to reflect on the sensory qualities of the session and use the opportunity to reminisce about sensory activities that they may have enjoyed in the past.
	To end the session, slowly brighten the room and return the conversation to everyday discussion.
Activity characteristics	There is no pressure to perform to a set of rules or achieve an end result. There is an element of creativity and spontaneity.

Details of multisensory activity: which pieces of equipment were selected and length of the session, any specific details regarding the caregiver's interaction with the person.

Activity plan: list other sensory activities that match a person's activity profile that can support this multisensory activity, e.g. food tasting, flower arranging.

QCS PAL ACTIVITY PROFILE FOR MULTISENSORY ENVIRONMENTS

SENSORY ACTIVITY LEVEL OF ABILITY

Name:. . . . .

Date:. . . . .

Likely abilities

- Is likely to respond to bodily sensations
- Can be guided to carry out single-step activities
- Can carry out more complex activities if they are broken down into one step at a time

Likely limitations

- May not have any conscious plan to carry out a movement to achieve a particular end result
- May be relying on others to make social contact

Caregiver's role

- To enable the person to experience the effect of the sensory activity on his/her senses
- To break the activity down into one step at a time
- To keep directions simple and understandable
- To approach and make first contact with the person

Using the PAL Activity Profile to support the person

Position of objects	Having established a sensory profile, select objects that target preferred senses. Stimulate the preferred senses first, then move on to those senses that receive little or no stimulus through everyday activity. Make sure the person is aware of the objects by making bodily contact.
Verbal directions	Reinforce any verbal directions with guided movements. Limit requests to carry out actions to the naming of the action and the multisensory object involved, e.g. 'lift your arm', 'hold the optic fibre'. Support these requests with guided movements if necessary. Use body language to help the person to settle and explore the object. If the person is new to multisensory objects, consider introducing the objects to them outside the room. Reinforce any verbal or non-verbal communication with positive affirmation, e.g. 'The optic fibres look like Christmas tree lights.'

Demonstrated directions and Working with others	Allow the person to settle in the room and explore any objects. Start with main room lights on and slowly dim the room. The session may last for up to 20 minutes, but end the session if the person is no longer able to concentrate on the task or if they fall asleep (this approach is designed to stimulate rather than relax).
	The ideal session should be one-to-one but a group of two may be accommodated.
	Break each activity down into one step at a time and limit the stimulus to no more than two of the objects operating at any one time. If the person appears distracted by the number of items operating, limit them to one.
	Allow the person to explore and handle the objects. Do not enforce any instructions on how to use or handle the objects unless the person is placing himself or herself in danger. Ensure that the person is able to access the sensory qualities of each object and use the opportunity to discuss how the sensory activity feels. Repeat the activity for as long as the person wishes to reinforce the sensory component. Draw the person's attention to the multisensory activity by the use of touch or by using the person's name.
	To end the session, slowly brighten the room and return the conversation to everyday discussion.
Activity characteristics	The activity is used as an opportunity for an enhanced sensory experience. Repetitive actions within this activity will reinforce the experience. The use of a multisensory environment will help reduce conflicting sensory stimuli and help focus attention and increase arousal levels.

Details of multisensory activity: which pieces of equipment were selected and length of the session, any specific details regarding the caregiver's interaction with the person.

Activity plan: list other sensory activities that match a person's activity profile that can support this multisensory activity, e.g. food tasting, hand massage, dancing.

QCS PAL ACTIVITY PROFILE FOR MULTISENSORY ENVIRONMENTS

REFLEX ACTIVITY LEVEL OF ABILITY

Name: . . . .

Date:. . . . .

Likely abilities

- Can make reflex responses to direct sensory stimulation
- Direct sensory stimulation can increase awareness of self and others
- May respond to social engagement through the use of body language

Likely limitations

- May not be aware of the surrounding environment or even their own body
- May have difficulty organizing the multiple sensations that are being experienced
- May become agitated in an environment that is over-stimulating

Caregiver's role

- To enable the person to be more aware of themselves
- To arouse the person to be more aware of their surroundings
- To engage the person through direct sensory stimulation
- To monitor the environment and reduce or control competing and multiple stimuli such as loud noises or background sounds

Using the PAL Activity Profile to support the person

Position of objects	Make available to the person objects that stimulate all of the senses (sight, sound, touch, taste, smell, movement). Directly stimulate the area of the body to be targeted, for example touching the palm of the hand/arms/feet, shining visual stimuli into the line of vision, placing aromas directly under the nose for olfactory stimulation. Ensure all the senses are stimulated equally. Look for signs that the person is aware of the objects, such as eye/head/hand movement, verbal responses, moving parts of their body.
Verbal directions	Help the person to settle and explore the objects. Guide all movements and reinforce with simple one-word verbal directions. Use a warm, reassuring tone and adapt volume to establish a connection with the person. If the person is new to the multisensory room ensure that they are settled with each object before exploring its sensory components. Maintain eye contact and reinforce the activity with appropriate body language and gestures.

✓

Demonstrated directions and Working with others	Bring the person into the room and settle them in a comfortable chair. If the person is in a wheelchair, transfer them to an easy chair. Start with main room lights on and slowly dim the room. The session may last for up to ten minutes, but end the session if the person is no longer able to concentrate on the task or if they fall asleep (this approach is designed to stimulate rather than relax). The session should be one-to-one. Break each activity down into one step at a time and limit the stimulus to one object operating at any one time. Repeat the activity for as long as the person is able to tolerate it. The activity is in direct response to the level of stimulation needed to arouse. Guide the person by touch to explore and handle the objects. Do not enforce any instructions on how to use or handle the objects unless the person is placing themselves in danger. Ensure that the person is able to access the sensory qualities of each object, and use your body language and tone of voice to enhance the level of stimulation. Maintain eye contact; make maximum use of facial expression, gestures and body postures for non-verbal communication. Use social actions that can be imitated such as smiling, waving, stroking. To end the session, slowly brighten the room and allow the person to become accustomed to the everyday environment. Adapt tone of voice and body language to the new environment.
Activity characteristics	This activity arouses conscious awareness of self and the immediate environment using the single senses of sight, sound, touch, taste, smell and movement.

Details of multisensory activity: which pieces of equipment were selected and length of the session, any specific details regarding the caregiver's interaction with the person.

Activity plan: list other sensory activities that match a person's activity profile that can support this multisensory activity, e.g. food tasting, hand massage, textured objects.

QCS PAL INDIVIDUAL ACTION PLAN: PLANNED LEVEL

Name: . . . .

Date:. . . . .

DRESSING SUPPORT AT A PLANNED LEVEL

Favourite garments

. . . .

Preferred routine

. . . .

. . . .

. . . .

Grooming likes and dislikes

. . . .

. . . .

. . . .

Method:

- Encourage the person to plan what to wear and to select own clothes from the wardrobe.
- Encourage the person to put on their own clothes; be available to assist if required.
- Point out labels on clothing to help orientate the back from the front.
- Encourage the person to attend to grooming such as brushing hair, putting on make-up, cleaning shoes.

Additional notes:

. . . .

. . . .

. . . .

. . . .

. . . .

✓

BATHING/SHOWERING SUPPORT AT A PLANNED LEVEL
Favourite toiletries

. . . .

Preferred routine

. . . .

. . . .

. . . .

Bathing likes and dislikes

. . . .

. . . .

. . . .

Method:

- Encourage the person to plan when they will have the bath, to draw the water or turn on the shower and to select toiletries from the usual cupboard or shelf.
- Encourage the person to wash their own body; be available to assist if required.
- Encourage the person to release the water afterwards or turn off the shower, and to wipe the bath/shower unit.

Additional notes:

. . . .

. . . .

. . . .

. . . .

. . . .

DINING SUPPORT AT A PLANNED LEVEL
Favourite foods

. . . .

Preferred routine

. . . .

. . . .

. . . .

Dining likes and dislikes

. . . .

. . . .

. . . .

Method:

- Encourage the person to select when and what they wish to eat.
- Encourage the person to prepare the dining table and to select the cutlery, crockery and condiments from the usual cupboards or drawers.
- Encourage the person to clear away afterwards.

Additional notes:

. . . .

. . . .

. . . .

. . . .

. . . .

QCS PAL INDIVIDUAL ACTION PLAN: EXPLORATORY LEVEL

Name: . . . .

Date:. . . . .

DRESSING SUPPORT AT AN EXPLORATORY LEVEL

Favourite garments

. . . .

Preferred routine

. . . .

. . . .

. . . .

Grooming likes and dislikes

. . . .

. . . .

. . . .

Method:

- Encourage discussion about the clothing to be worn for the day: is it suitable for the weather or the occasion? Is it a favourite item?
- Spend time colour-matching items of clothing and select accessories.
- Break down the activity into manageable chunks: help lay the clothes out in order so that underclothing is at the top of the pile. If the person wishes to be helped, talk the person through the task: 'Put on your underclothes'; 'Now put on your trousers/dress and shirt/cardigan.'
- Encourage the person to check their appearance in the mirror.

Additional notes:

. . . .

. . . .

. . . .

. . . .

. . . .

BATHING/SHOWERING SUPPORT AT AN EXPLORATORY LEVEL

Favourite toiletries

. . . .

Preferred routine

. . . .

. . . .

. . . .

Bathing likes and dislikes

. . . .

. . . .

. . . .

Method

- Break down the activity into manageable chunks: suggest that the person fills the bath or turns on the shower. When that is accomplished suggest that they gather together items such as soap, shampoo, flannel and towels.
- When the person is in the bath/shower suggest that they soap and rinse their upper body. When that is accomplished suggest that they soap and rinse their lower body.
- Ensure that bathing/showering items are on view and that containers are clearly labelled.
- Have attractive objects around the bathroom such as unusual bath oil bottles or shells and encourage discussion and exploration of them.

Additional notes:

. . . .

. . . .

. . . .

. . . .

. . . .

DINING SUPPORT AT AN EXPLORATORY LEVEL

Favourite foods

. . . .

Preferred routine

. . . .

. . . .

. . . .

✓

Dining likes and dislikes

. . . .

. . . .

. . . .

Method

- Store cutlery and crockery in view and encourage the person to select their own tools for dining.
- Offer food using simple choices.
- Create a social atmosphere using table decorations and music, and promote conversation.

Additional notes:

. . . .

. . . .

. . . .

. . . .

. . . .

QCS PAL INDIVIDUAL ACTION PLAN: SENSORY LEVEL

Name: . . . .

Date: . . . .

DRESSING SUPPORT AT A SENSORY LEVEL

Favourite garments

. . . .

Preferred routine

. . . .

. . . .

. . . .

Grooming likes and dislikes

. . . .

. . . .

. . . .

Method

- Offer a simple choice of clothing to be worn.
- Spend a few moments enjoying the sensations of the clothing: feeling the fabric, gently rubbing the person's hand over different textures, or smelling the clean laundry.
- Break down the task into one step at a time: 'Put on your vest'; 'Now put on your pants'; 'Now put on your stockings'; 'Now put on your dress.'

Additional notes:

. . . .

. . . .

. . . .

. . . .

. . . .

✓

BATHING/SHOWERING SUPPORT AT A SENSORY LEVEL
Favourite toiletries

. . . .

Preferred routine

. . . .

. . . .

. . . .

Bathing likes and dislikes

. . . .

. . . .

. . . .

Method

- Prepare the bathroom and run the bath water for the person.
- Make the bathroom warm and inviting – play music, use scented oils or bubble bath, have candles lit on a safely out-of-reach shelf.
- Break down the task into one step at a time and give the person simple directions: 'Rub the soap on the cloth'; 'Rub your arm'; 'Rinse your arm'; 'Rub your chest'; 'Rinse your chest.'

Additional notes:

. . . .

. . . .

. . . .

. . . .

. . . .

DINING SUPPORT AT A SENSORY LEVEL
Favourite foods

. . . .

Preferred routine

. . . .

. . . .

. . . .

Dining likes and dislikes

· ·

· ·

· ·

Method

- Serve food so that it presents a variety of colours, tastes and textures.
- Offer the person finger foods, encourage them to feel the food.
- Offer the person a spoon, place it in their hand and direct them to 'Scoop the potato'; 'Lift your arm'; 'Open your mouth.'
- Provide hand-under-hand support to start the movement from plate to mouth, if needed.

Additional notes:

· ·

· ·

· ·

· ·

· ·

QCS PAL INDIVIDUAL ACTION PLAN: REFLEX LEVEL

Name:. . . . .

Date:. . . . .

DRESSING SUPPORT AT A REFLEX LEVEL

Favourite garments

. . . .

Preferred routine

. . . .

. . . .

. . . .

Grooming likes and dislikes

. . . .

. . . .

. . . .

Method

- Prepare the clothing for the person, ensure the dressing area is private and that a chair or bed at the right height is available for sitting.
- Talk through each stage of the activity as you put the clothing on the person. Use a calm tone, speak slowly and smile to indicate that you are non-threatening.
- Stimulate a response in the limb being dressed by using firm but gentle stroking. Ask the person to assist you when necessary by using one-word requests: 'Lift', 'Stand', 'Sit'.
- At the end of dressing, spend some time brushing the person's hair using firm massaging brush strokes.

Additional notes:

. . . .

. . . .

. . . .

. . . .

. . . .

BATHING/SHOWERING SUPPORT AT A REFLEX LEVEL

Favourite toiletries

. . . .

Preferred routine

. . . .

. . . .

. . . .

Bathing likes and dislikes

. . . .

. . . .

. . . .

Method

- Prepare the bathroom and run the bath water for the person, put in scented bath products (lavender will aid relaxation).
- Ensure that the bathroom is warm and inviting, and feels secure by closing the door and curtains and providing a slip-resistant bath mat in the bath and on the floor. Clear away any unnecessary items which may be confusing.
- Use firm, massaging movements when soaping and rinsing the person.
- Wrap them securely in a towel when they are out of the bath.

Additional notes:

. . . .

. . . .

. . . .

. . . .

. . . .

DINING SUPPORT AT A REFLEX LEVEL

Favourite foods

. . . .

Preferred routine

. . . .

. . . .

. . . .

Dining likes and dislikes

. . . .

. . . .

. . . .

Method

- Use touch on the person's forearm to make contact, maintain eye contact, and smile to indicate the pleasure of the activity.
- Place a spoon in the person's hand. Close your hand over the person's and raise the spoon with food on it to their mouth.
- As the food reaches the person's mouth say 'open' and open your own mouth to demonstrate. Touch the person's lips gently with the spoon.

Additional notes:

. . . .

. . . .

. . . .

. . . .

. . . .

QCS POOL ACTIVITY LEVEL (PAL) ENGAGEMENT MEASURE

Name of patient/service user:

. . . .

Date completed:

. . . .

Activity engaged in:

. . . .

Completed by:

. . . .

		DATE				NOT OBSERVED DURING ACTIVITY (0 points)	OBSERVED AT TIMES BUT NOT CONSISTENTLY (1 point)	ENGAGED CONSISTENTLY IN KEEPING WITH THE ACTIVITY (2 points)
COGNITIVE ABILITIES	Goal aware					Has an end result in mind, can plan how to achieve this and can work towards this		
	Initiates					Independently starts an action toward another person or object		
	Attends					Notices and focuses on a sensation		
	Concentrates					Sustains attention on the activity, person or object		
	Adjusts					Adapts actions to meet the demands of the activity		
	Explores					Shows interest in and seeks to engage with environment and objects		
	Responds					Reacts to sensations, verbal requests or prompts		
PHYSICAL ABILITIES	Stabilizes					Maintains balance and posture while moving, standing or sitting		
	Coordinates					Moves smoothly while negotiating obstacles or handling objects		
	Manipulates					Uses tools and objects to achieve an end result. Handles an object in response to the sensation it generates		
	Grips objects					Uses appropriate strength to hold objects securely		
	Releases objects					Independently and appropriately lets go of objects		
SOCIAL INTERACTION	Aware of others					Notices and responds directly or indirectly to the presence of others		
	Shares objects					Offers and accepts objects to/from others		
	Vocal interactions					Uses vocal sounds to make a connection with others		
	Non-vocal interactions					Uses body language to make a connection with others		

EMOTIONAL WELL-BEING	Hope					Has a sense of meaning and positivity to the activity
	Agency					Has a sense of purposefulness during the activity
	Self-confidence					Has a sense of empowerment and autonomy when carrying out the activity
	Self-esteem					Has a sense of fulfilment when carrying out and on completion of the activity
	TOTAL					

COMPLETING THE ENGAGEMENT MEASURE

1. Use one Engagement Measure sheet for each personal care or leisure activity that you wish to record for the person.
2. Complete one of the five columns to record one event of the activity.
3. Decide the frequency of the recording: for example, it could be weekly, fortnightly or monthly.
4. Record the abilities in each cell of the column with a numerical score as shown in the key: zero for not observed during the activity; one point for observed but not consistently; and two points for engaged consistently in keeping with the activity.
5. You can also colour code your entries on the sheet with red for zero, yellow for one and green for two points.
6. Use the scores and/or the colours to monitor the impact of your support to the person.
7. If you notice that there has been a significant change in the cognitive abilities or the social interaction of the person, complete another PAL Checklist.
8. If you notice that there has been a significant change in physical abilities or emotional well-being, you may need to refer the person for a medical assessment.

Chapter 2

INTRODUCTION TO PART 1

USING THIS GUIDE

The QCS PAL Instrument is based on the underpinning principle that people with cognitive impairment also have abilities and that when an enabling environment is presented to the person, these potential abilities can be realized. Occupation is the key to unlocking this potential. In order to present an occupation to the person with cognitive impairment so that they can engage with it, their impairments and abilities must first be understood. In addition, an individual is motivated to engage in occupations that have personal significance. Therefore an understanding of what drives the person, using information about their unique biography and about personality, is also vital. The QCS PAL Instrument provides the user with the means to collect this important information and to use it to compile an individual profile that aids in the presentation of occupations to the person.

The QCS PAL Instrument comprises:

- Life History Profile
- Checklist describing the way that an individual engages in occupations
- Activity Profile with general information for engaging the person in a range of meaningful occupations
- Individual Action Plan that includes directions for facilitating the engagement of the person in activities of daily living
- Engagement Measure that provides a record over time of an individual's cognitive, physical and social abilities and their state of well-being during engagement in a specific activity.

A blank copy of the QCS PAL Instrument is provided in Chapter 1 of this book and may be photocopied for manual use by readers with people with cognitive impairment. The digital version of the QCS PAL Instrument can be freely downloaded at www.qcs.co.uk/digital-pool-activity-level-pal-instrument. This digital version will automatically calculate the abilities of the individual from the completed checklist to create the PAL Guide which is a comprehensive combined version of this book-based PAL Activity Profile and the PAL Individual Action Plan.

THEORETICAL BACKGROUND

The QCS PAL Instrument draws from several models of understanding human behaviour: the Lifespan Approach to human development; the Dialectical Model of a person-centred approach to the interplay of social, neurological and psychological factors; and the Functional Information Processing Model.

THE LIFESPAN APPROACH TO HUMAN DEVELOPMENT

Theorists of human development propose that individuals' physical, intellectual, social and emotional skills change over time, according to the experiences they encounter. When this process is viewed in this way it is termed the Lifespan Approach. The first major theorist to acknowledge the lifelong nature of human development was Erik Erikson (Atkinson, Atkinson and Hilgard 1983) who described the 'eight Ages of Man', each of which presents the individual with a new developmental task to be worked on. Erikson proposed that human development does not end when physical maturity is reached, but that it is a continuous process from birth through to old age. His eight stages were based on the belief that the psychological development of an individual depends on the social relations they experience at various points in life. When working with people with cognitive impairment it is helpful not only to recognize the importance of this cradle-to-grave development theory, but also to understand some of the developmental processes which take place in infancy and childhood. A more detailed description of developmental theory can be found elsewhere, but a brief description of neurological development is included here in order to clarify the theory underpinning the QCS PAL Instrument.

When a child is born, the higher part of the brain is like a blank page waiting to be written on as experiences are encountered. The higher part of the brain is concerned with cognition, which includes functions such as thought, judgement, comprehension and reasoning. It also controls complex functions such as processing information from the environment sent from the sensory organs – the eyes, ears, nose, mouth and skin – via the nervous system to the brain. Infants learn from these experiences which are 'written on' to the higher brain as memories in the form of patterns of nerve connections. This enables infants to judge new experiences against previous ones and to make decisions about how to respond. They also begin to be able to adapt to new situations as they arise by matching the experience to similar ones. It is a function of the higher brain to interpret information and to decide on the necessary action.

At first, the new-born baby is relying on the more primitive underlying part of the brain, which is concerned with basic emotions and needs. This primitive brain is responsible for early behaviour such as fear of strangers, and the forming of a bond or specific attachment with another person. It also causes individuals, throughout their life, to experience and communicate social and emotional nuances (via emotional speech, laughing, crying, expressing sympathy, compassion), and to desire to form and maintain an emotional attachment. The primitive brain therefore enables us to be what is essentially a person: to establish the identity and existence that is conferred on us through contact with others.

THE DIALECTICAL MODEL OF A PERSON-CENTRED APPROACH

This model was first proposed by Tom Kitwood when exploring factors other than the neurological impairment that combine to cause the disability of dementia. It has now become the underpinning value-base for dementia care. One way of viewing these factors is as an equation where: $D = P + B + H + NI + SP$ (Kitwood 1993). This is a simple way of showing that any individual's dementia (D) is the result of a complex interaction between five main components: personality (P), biography (B), health (H), neurological impairment (NI) and social psychology (SP). To view dementia only as a result of the neurological impairment caused by the medical picture of Alzheimer's disease, for example, would be to view an incomplete picture. An individual's personality and life history will colour and shape the picture, although these will have largely been developed and are unchangeable.

Physical and mental ill-health often causes people to behave differently, as they try to cope with feelings of pain or discomfort. Some people with neurological impairments are unable to communicate their needs to others verbally. Their behaviour, which is another form of communication, can be misinterpreted as part of their condition, and the inappropriate response from others contributes further to the disability of the individual.

The final component of social psychology in the equation is viewed as the one that can have the most significant impact, either for better or worse. This is how the effects of meetings with others can have an impact on the emotional state of the person and either add to the disability of the person by undermining skills and causing feelings of ill-being, or reduce the disability by creating an environment that is empowering to the person and nurtures well-being.

A person-centred philosophy, therefore, recognizes the uniqueness of the person more than their impairment. However, all of the factors that combine within the person need to be understood so that disability is minimized or avoided. Relationships are felt to be at the heart of person-centred philosophy, and positive contacts with others can ensure the well-being of people with dementia, regardless of the level of impairment.

Well-being can be described as the state of having a sense of hope, agency, self-confidence and self-esteem. Hope in this way refers to a sense of expectation of positive experiences. Agency refers to a sense of having an impact on the surrounding environment and of being able to make things happen. Self-confidence refers to the feeling of assurance in one's own ability. Self-esteem is a feeling of self-worth. The human need for occupation is satisfied when engagement in it also nurtures these states of well-being.

THE FUNCTIONAL INFORMATION PROCESSING MODEL

Cognition is the process by which we think and understand. When a person has a cognitive impairment, it may have one or more of several possible causes: illness, trauma, congenital differences or emotional stress. In all cases, there is damage to the nerve and brain tissue, most commonly in the higher brain. This damage causes cognitive impairments of judgement, reasoning, thinking and planning, which in turn can lead to disability such as dementia or learning disability. This will be the case if the physical and social environment is disempowering rather than compensating the person for their impairment or enabling them to adapt.

The Functional Information Processing Model is a model whose clinical application is grounded in occupational therapy (Pool 2011). Claudia K. Allen, an American occupational therapist, developed the model during her observations of clients with psychiatric disorders. The original theoretical base was influenced by Piaget's theory that cognitive development is a stage process (Piaget 1952). The cognitive model proposed by Piaget looks at the processes of human memory and puts great emphasis on aspects of being that require highly developed mental skills, but gives little consideration to feelings, emotions and relationships. Allen's later work (Allen 1999) has developed the theoretical base to include the work of Soviet psychologist Vygotsky, who proposed that human development is a social process involving close interactions between the child and its parents, and later its peers and teachers (Vygotsky 1978).

Allen's description of cognitive disability, based on these earlier theoretical bases, proposes that 'a restriction in voluntary motor action originating in the physical and chemical structures of the brain will produce observable limitations in routine task behaviour' (Allen 1985, p.31). Therefore, observing an individual's ability to carry out tasks can indicate damage to those structures. This is because the cognitive processes driving the motor actions in order for the task to be carried out are impaired.

Allen organized this evidence of cognitive impairment into six levels, using descriptions of how an individual attends to the environment, sensory cues and to objects. These cognitive levels, which measure a person's ability to function, are based on the stages of development proposed by Piaget. By identifying the cognitive disability of an individual, occupational therapists can also identify their remaining abilities. The occupational therapist's role is to then design and test activity environments that utilize these abilities, and to instruct others in maintaining those environments.

Functional cognition encompasses the complex and dynamic interactions between an individual's cognitive abilities and the activity context that produces observable performance. The QCS PAL Instrument Checklist identifies a person's overall cognitive functional level from Allen's levels from 0.8 to 5.8 by describing the person's ability to engage in nine functional domains. As with Allen's model, the PAL domain descriptions are based on cognitive development theory (Piaget 1952; Vygotsky 1978), with each domain providing four descriptions that are aligned to the executive function stages of these theorists. The PAL levels are: Planned, Exploratory, Sensory and Reflex, and the relationship between these and Allen's levels are presented in Table 2.1 (Pool 2022).

The QCS PAL Instrument takes the information from Allen's Functional Information Processing Model and presents it in a form that is accessible to those without an occupational therapy qualification. It provides the user with a self-interpreting assessment in the form of guides for creating and maintaining facilitating environments. The PAL further develops Allen's more recent attention to the importance of social connections in occupational performance, building on Vygotsky's insights into the importance of providing appropriate assistance and support to the individual while they engage in an activity. The PAL Instrument also combines the Functional Information Processing Model with the Socio-Psychological Model by focusing the user on the biography of the individual, and using this information as a guide to facilitating activities that are meaningful to them.

Table 2.1: PAL levels description with relationship to Allen's cognitive levels

PAL levels Allen's cognitive levels	REFLEX 1.0–1.8	SENSORY 2.0–3.4	EXPLORATORY 3.5–4.8	PLANNED 5.0–5.8
Likely abilities	Can make reflex responses to direct sensory stimulation.	Is likely to be responding to bodily sensations.	Can carry out very familiar activities in familiar surroundings.	Can explore different ways of carrying out an activity.
Likely limitations	May not be aware of the surrounding environment or even their own body.	May not have any conscious plan to carry out a movement to achieve a particular end result.	May not have an end result in mind when starting activities.	May not be able to solve problems that arise.

Caregiver's role	To enable the person to be more aware of themselves.	To enable the person to experience the effect of the activity on their senses.	To enable the person to experience the sensation of doing the activity rather than focusing on the end result.	To enable the person to take control of the activity and master the steps involved.

REFERENCES

Allen, C.K. (1985) *Occupational Therapy for Psychiatric Diseases: Measurement and Management of Cognitive Disabilities*. Boston, MA: Little, Brown.

Allen, C.K. (1999) *Structures of the Cognitive Performance Modes*. Ormond Beach, FL: Allen Conferences, Inc.

Atkinson, R.L., Atkinson, R.C. and Hilgard, E.R. (1983) *Introduction to Psychology (International Edition)*. New York, NY: Harcourt Brace Jovanovich.

Kitwood, T. (1993) 'Discover the person not the disease.' *Journal of Dementia Care*, 1(1), 16–17.

Piaget, J. (1952) *The Origins of Intelligence in Children*. New York, NY: International Universities Press.

Pool, J. (2011) 'The Functional Information Processing Model.' In E. Duncan (ed.) *Occupational Therapy* (fifth edition). Edinburgh: Elsevier Churchill Livingstone.

Pool, J. (2022) 'The Pool Activity Level (PAL) Instrument – An Occupational Focus for Engagement, Function and Well-being.' In F. Maclean, A. Warren, E. Hunter and L. Westcott (eds) *Occupational Therapy for Dementia*. London: Jessica Kingsley Publishers.

Vygotsky, L.S. (1978) *The Development of Higher Psychological Processes*. Boston, MA: Harvard University Press.

Chapter 3

THE FOUR ACTIVITY LEVELS

Completing the PAL Checklist enables caregivers to recognize the ability of a person with cognitive impairment to engage in activity. Any individual who knows the person well, by considering how they generally function when carrying out activities, particularly those involving other people, can complete it. These observations should have been made in several situations over a period of two weeks. If the person lives in a group setting, such as a care home, the observations should be a compilation from all involved caregivers, including activity providers, care staff and ancillary staff. In this way, the variation of abilities and disabilities, which can occur in an individual over a period of time, is taken into account, and an occupational profile can be made. The PAL Activity Profile gives an overview of the way that a person best engages in activities and how to create a facilitating and enabling environment.

Because there are many factors affecting an individual's ability to engage in an activity – cognitive integrity, the meaningfulness of the task, the familiarity of the environment, the support of others – it is likely that an individual will reveal a variation in their level of ability in different activities. The QCS PAL Instrument acknowledges the importance of this and provides the opportunity to create an Individual Action Plan that allows for a varying degree of support in some of the personal activities of daily living.

The PAL is organized into four activity levels: *planned*, *exploratory*, *sensory* and *reflex*.

PLANNED ACTIVITY LEVEL

At a *planned* activity level the person can work towards completing an activity, but may not be able to solve any problems that arise while in the process. They will be able to look in obvious places for objects needed, but may not be able to search beyond the usual places. Caregivers assisting someone at this level will need to keep their sentences short, and avoid using words like 'and' or 'but' which tend to be used to link two sentences together into a more complex one. Caregivers will also need to stand by to help solve any problems should they arise. People functioning at a planned activity level are able to carry out activities that achieve a tangible result.

EXPLORATORY ACTIVITY LEVEL

At an *exploratory* activity level the person can carry out very familiar tasks in familiar surroundings. However, at this level people are most concerned with the effect of doing the activity rather than the consequence, and may not have an end result in mind. Therefore, a creative and spontaneous approach by caregivers to activities is helpful. If an activity involves more than two or three steps, a person at this level will need help in breaking the activity into manageable chunks. Directions need to be made very simple and the use of memory aids such as task lists, calendars and labelling of frequently used items can be very helpful.

SENSORY ACTIVITY LEVEL

At a *sensory* activity level the person may not have many thoughts or ideas about carrying out an activity; they are mainly concerned with sensation and with moving their body in response to those sensations. People at this level can be guided to carry out single-step tasks such as sweeping or winding wool. More complex activities can only be carried out when directed one step at a time. Therefore, caregivers need to ensure that the person at this activity level has the opportunity to experience a wide variety of sensations, and to carry out one-step tasks. Directions to maximize this opportunity need to be kept very simple and be reinforced by demonstrating the action required.

REFLEX ACTIVITY LEVEL

A person at a *reflex* activity level may not be aware of the surrounding environment or even of their own body. They are living in a subliminal or sub-conscious state, where movement is a reflex response to a stimulus. Therefore, people wishing to enter into this person's consciousness need to use direct sensory stimulation. If direct stimulation is used, the person's self-awareness can be raised. A person at this level may have difficulty in organizing more than one sensation which is being experienced at the same time. Excessive or multiple stimuli can cause distress, so crowds, loud noises and background clamour should be avoided. Activities at this level should focus on introducing a single sensation to the person. Caregivers interacting with a person at a *reflex* activity level need to use all their communication skills to enter into the world of the person. Language skills tend to play only a minor role and should be kept to single-word directions, although the use of facial expression and of a warm and reassuring tone and volume can be vital in establishing a communication channel.

Chapter 4

RELIABILITY AND VALIDITY OF THE PAL CHECKLIST

Jennifer Wenborn, David Challis and Martin Orrell

INTRODUCTION

Development of the QCS PAL Instrument is outlined at the beginning of this book. It is now used in a variety of service settings for older people with dementia care throughout the UK and beyond. General opinion obtained through professional networks suggested that it is a useful and practical tool. Indeed, it is recommended in the national clinical guideline for dementia (NICE 2006) as an instrument to guide providers of daily living and leisure activities. This acknowledges that in order for care staff to integrate occupational opportunities into their daily care provision, they need a quick and easy-to-use assessment tool. Assessment tools do need to be 'fit for purpose', and this can be demonstrated by assessing their psychometric properties (the technical construction and qualities of the instrument) (Bowling 2002), to ensure that they are valid and reliable for use, both in practice and in research.

AIM OF THE STUDY

The aim of this study was to assess the validity and reliability of the PAL Checklist when used with older people who have dementia.

METHOD

Study design

There were two phases to the study. Phase one used a postal questionnaire to assess content validity. Phase two assessed the criterion, concurrent and construct validity; internal consistency; and inter-rater and test–retest reliability in a sample of older people with dementia.

Validity

Validity refers to how well an instrument assesses the concept that it is intended to assess (Bowling 2002). In this case, the concept is the individual's cognitive level of ability to engage in activity. Several aspects of validity can be measured. Content validity considers the extent to which the instrument assesses the scope of the concept. It is commonly measured by consulting experts in the field and professionals, users and carers relevant to the area.

Other aspects of validity, such as criterion, concurrent and construct validity, can be measured by comparing the performance of the instrument, alongside other relevant assessments, with a group of participants from the target population, in this case older people with dementia.

Reliability

Reliability considers how consistent the instrument is (Bowling 2002). There are three aspects. Internal consistency refers to how the results obtained for each test item correlate with each other. Inter-rater reliability refers to the test's consistency when used by different assessors. Test–retest reliability looks at how far the results are consistent when the test is repeated (e.g. a week later). Assuming the clinical picture has not changed, then if the test is reliable, the results would be very similar.

Phase one – content validity

A postal questionnaire was sent to three groups: (a) the Royal College of Occupational Therapists Specialist Section: Older People's Dementia Clinical Forum; (b) the National Association for Providers of Activities for Older People (NAPA); and (c) other experts, mainly occupational therapists and activity providers. The questionnaire asked respondents to indicate their professional background using the following options: occupational therapist, occupational therapy (OT) assistant/technician, activity provider, care assistant, nurse, doctor, psychologist, social worker, other (please specify). Respondents were asked if they had previously used the PAL Checklist, and if so, in what type of setting: ward/day service/person's home/care home? The following questions were asked: 'Are any important items missing?'; 'Are any items redundant?'; 'Are the instructions clear?'

Each of these questions required the respondent to circle either 'yes' or 'no' and space was provided for further comment or explanation. Respondents were asked, 'How easy or difficult do you think it is to complete the PAL Checklist?', and given four options to choose from: very difficult/quite difficult/quite easy/very easy. Finally, respondents were asked to rank the importance of each of the nine checklist items using a four-point scale, when 1 = not important; 2 = quite important; 3 = very important; and 4 = essential. The number of responses to each item in the questionnaire was counted, and the percentages calculated for each category.

Phase two – validity and reliability

A sample of 60 older people with dementia was recruited from a range of in-patient, day hospital and continuing care services provided within a mental health trust. Participants had to: be aged 60 years or over; have received the service for at least two weeks (or four visits in the case of day hospitals); meet the criteria often used to diagnose dementia (American Psychiatric Association 1994); and score less than 24 on the Mini Mental State Examination (MMSE) (Folstein, Folstein and McHugh 1975). Information sheets explaining the study were provided and, if possible, consent was obtained directly from participants. For those people who were not able to sign a consent form, their potential participation was discussed either with their relatives (if applicable) and/or a relevant member of staff, for example their keyworker, in order to protect their best interests. Participants' general practitioners were informed that they were taking part in the study. The NHS Barking and Havering Local Research Ethics Committee provided ethical approval (reference number: 05/Q0602/8).

INSTRUMENTS

The Pool Activity Level (PAL) Checklist (Pool 2002)

Please see Chapter 1 for the complete QCS PAL Instrument, including the Checklist. The following package of instruments was also used in the study.

Mini Mental State Examination (MMSE) (Folstein *et al.* 1975)

The MMSE is a well-known cognitive screening test frequently used in clinical and research settings. Validity, test–retest and inter-rater reliability were established by the original authors (Folstein *et al.* 1975) and have been further reviewed by Tombaugh and McIntyre (1992). The maximum score of 30 indicates no cognitive impairment. It was predicted that higher MMSE scores would correlate with higher PAL activity levels.

Clinical Dementia Rating (CDR) Scale (Hughes *et al.* 1982)

The CDR is a global rating of the severity of dementia. Inter-rater reliability has been established (Berg, Miller and Storandt 1988; Hughes *et al.* 1982). The chronic care version includes two further categories of severity: profound and terminal. It was therefore used in this study to cover the range of service settings included. The lowest possible score of 0 indicates no evidence of dementia and a score of 5 indicates the most severe level. It was predicted that lower CDR scores would correlate with higher PAL activity levels.

Barthel Index (BI) (Mahoney and Barthel 1965)

The BI measures functional ability and the degree of assistance required (physical and/or verbal) in ten daily living activities. The score indicates the individual's level of dependency. Validity, inter-rater and test–retest reliability and sensitivity have been assessed as being excellent (Wade and Collin 1988). The activities assessed by both the BI and the PAL Checklist are: bathing/washing, getting dressed, eating. The maximum score of 100 indicates independence in daily living activities. It was predicted that higher BI scores would correlate with higher PAL activity levels.

Bristol Activities of Daily Living Scale (BADLS) (Bucks *et al.* 1996)

The BADLS is a carer-rated scale comprising 20 items. It was developed specifically for use with people with dementia. Face, construct and concurrent validity, and test–retest reliability, have been confirmed (Bucks *et al.* 1996). The activities assessed by both the BADLS and the PAL Checklist are: bathing/washing, dressing, eating, communication and participation in activities. The lowest possible score of 0 indicates independence in daily living activities, while the highest possible score of 60 indicates maximum dependence. It was predicted that lower BADLS scores would correlate with higher PAL activity levels.

Clifton Assessment Procedures for the Elderly – Behaviour Rating Scale (CAPE–BRS) (Pattie and Gilleard 1979)

The CAPE–BRS is a carer-rated scale that assesses a range of daily living activities and behaviours, with the aim of indicating the individual's level of dependency. Four subsections consider: physical dependency, apathy, communication difficulties and social disturbance. The activities assessed by both the CAPE–BRS and the PAL Checklist are: bathing, dressing, participation in activity, socializing and communication. The lowest possible score of 0 indicates independent function, while the highest possible score of 36 indicates maximum dependency. It was predicted that lower CAPE–BRS scores would correlate with higher PAL activity levels.

ASSESSING VALIDITY

Three raters, all occupational therapists working within the NHS Trust, collected the data using the following process. The MMSE was completed with the participant with dementia. A member of staff was interviewed about each participant and asked to complete the PAL Checklist. Their observations of how the individual had actually behaved over the previous two weeks, plus information obtained from the individual's care plan, enabled the rater to complete the other instruments: CDR, BI, BADLS, CAPE–BRS.

Criterion validity was assessed by comparing the PAL activity levels by service setting. It had been predicted that the participants who were attending a day hospital, that is, they were still living in the community, would achieve a higher PAL activity level than those living in continuing care.

Construct validity was evaluated using an inter-item correlation matrix. It had been anticipated that the highest correlation would be within two groups of activities. The first group comprised: bathing, dressing, practical activities, use of objects and looking at a newspaper; these all rely on being able to recognize and use objects appropriately and in the correct sequence. The second group comprised: contact with others, groupwork and communication; these all depend on interacting and communicating with other people.

Concurrent validity was measured by correlating the PAL Checklist results with the test scores obtained using the other instruments. There is no relevant 'gold standard' instrument against which to directly compare the PAL Checklist, that is, a generic, quick and easy-to-use tool that assesses an individual's level of ability to engage in activities. The other instruments were therefore selected because they either assess key factors that influence the ability to engage in activity, such as the severity of dementia (CDR) and degree of cognitive impairment (MMSE), or they assess the ability to carry out specific activities that are also assessed by the PAL Checklist (BI, BADLS, CAPE–BRS).

ASSESSING RELIABILITY

Inter-rater reliability was measured by asking a second member of staff to complete the PAL Checklist on the same day, without discussing or comparing the results. Test–retest reliability was measured by asking the same member of staff to complete the PAL Checklist again about a week later.

RESULTS

Phase one

A total of 122 questionnaires were circulated, and 102 completed questionnaires were received, which represents a response rate of 84 per cent. Fifty-five respondents (54%) had previously used the PAL Checklist and 47 (46%) had not. Of those who had used the instrument, 25 (45%) had used it in a ward; 20 (36%) in a day service; 22 (40%) in a person's own home; and 27 (49%) in a care home setting. Seventy-five (74%) were occupational therapists or occupational therapy support workers; 12 (12%) were activity providers; and the other 14 (14%) were from a variety of professional backgrounds, including nursing and psychology.

CONTENT VALIDITY

Ninety-five (97%) said the instructions for completing the PAL Checklist were clear. Using a four-point scale ranging from very difficult to very easy, 90 respondents (93%) rated the PAL Checklist as quite easy or very easy to complete. Seven items were ranked as very important or essential by at least 73 respondents (77%). The most highly ranked of these seven items was contact with others, by 93 (99%) of the respondents. This was followed by: communication skills, 89 (94%); eating, 87 (93%); getting dressed, 79 (84%); bathing/washing, 78 (82%); use of objects, 74 (78%); and practical activities, 73 (77%). Fifty-seven (60%) ranked groupwork skills as very important or essential, and a further 33 (35%) ranked it as quite important. Only 30 respondents (32%) ranked the newspaper item as very important or essential, but a further 45 (47%) ranked it as quite important. Most respondents (48, or 55%) said that no important items were missing. Although 39 (45%) said that one or more important items were missing, and 52 (60%) made comments, there was no consistent pattern to their responses. Nine responses (17%) related to describing the individual's mood and motivation; for example: 'perhaps "mood" or "ability to cooperate" could be included?' Eight (15%) commented on the individual's level of orientation and/or ability to navigate the environment; for example: 'orientation to place, e.g. ability to find way around familiar/unfamiliar buildings or places'. Five responses (10%) suggested the inclusion of mobility and another five (10%) felt that 'having information and assessment of a person's ability to transfer, i.e. on and off bed, chair and toilet' was needed. A further five (10%) specifically suggested that using the toilet and/or continence should be included.

Twenty-four respondents (27%) felt that there were some redundant items. Their comments related mainly to two items: 'groupwork' (13, or 15%) and 'looking at a newspaper' (14, or 16%), and were based on the practitioner's own experience of using the instrument. The difficulty of completing the groupwork item when assessing people living on their own in the community was highlighted. Its relevance was also questioned, as this approach is not seen as appropriate for those in the later stages of dementia. It was also pointed out that 'groupwork is the kind of skill which has something to do with staff'. There were three themes related to the newspaper item: some felt that it could be difficult to assess; others that it might not be a familiar activity to some people, and therefore not relevant to assess; while others stated, 'it is very specific', suggesting that 'this may be better widened to include other similar activities, such as TV'.

Phase two

Data was collected for 60 people with dementia. There were 20 from each of the following service settings: day hospital, in-patient ward and continuing care. The ratio of male to female participants was one to four. The participants' ages ranged from 64 to 96, with a mean (average) age of 78 years. Twenty (33%) lived in continuing care. The social situation of the remaining 40 people, when not in hospital, was as follows: 16 (40%) lived alone; 18 (45%) lived with a spouse or relative; and 6 (15%) lived in supported accommodation. The MMSE scores ranged from 0 to 22, with a mean score of 9. Fifty-five staff were interviewed to enable completion of the instruments. Their length of experience of working with older people with dementia ranged from 10 months to 27 years. Twenty-eight (51%) had a professional qualification (primarily registered mental nurse). Twelve (22%) had an NVQ or equivalent level qualification and the other 15 (27%) had no formal qualification.

CRITERION VALIDITY

The frequency of the PAL activity levels and each checklist item within each of the service settings is shown in Table 4.1. The frequency of PAL activity levels for the total sample (60) was 18 (30%) at planned activity level, 11 (18%) at exploratory activity level, 12 (20%) at sensory activity level and 19 (32%) at reflex activity level. Table 4.1 demonstrates that, as predicted, the day hospital attendees achieved higher PAL activity levels, which indicates a higher level of ability than those requiring the additional support provided within a continuing care setting. Conversely, those in continuing care obtained lower PAL activity levels, thus reflecting their higher level of dependency.

Table 4.1: Frequency (%) of PAL activity levels and PAL Checklist items per service setting (n=60)

PAL activity level	Day hospital	In-patient	Continuing care
Planned	11 (55%)	4 (20%)	3 (15%)
Exploratory	3 (15%)	5 (25%)	3 (15%)
Sensory	5 (25%)	7 (35%)	0 (0%)
Reflex	1 (5%)	4 (20%)	14 (70%)

CONCURRENT VALIDITY

Concurrent validity was demonstrated through correlating the PAL checklist scores with scores on the other instruments, using Spearman's rank order correlation coefficient (rho). The rho values for each correlation were as follows: MMSE (–0.75); BI (–0.71); CAPE–BRS (0.71); BADLS (0.82); and CDR (0.81).

A minimum value of 0.7 is recommended, and the nearer the value is to 1.0, the stronger is the correlation. All correlations were therefore highly significant ($p < 0.001$). As expected, the (negative) correlation with the MMSE and BI reflected that higher scores obtained using these tools indicate higher levels of cognitive ability and independence in daily living activities respectively and therefore correlate with higher PAL activity levels. Conversely, the (positive) correlation with the CAPE–BRS, BADLS and CDR reflects that higher scores obtained using these tools indicate higher dependency, poorer ability to perform daily living activities, and more severe dementia respectively – and so correlate with lower PAL activity levels.

CONSTRUCT VALIDITY

The correlation between each item of the PAL Checklist is shown in Table 4.2. In terms of convergent validity, again using Spearman's rank order correlation coefficient (rho), the highest correlations were found between practical activities and the use of objects (0.81), dressing (0.80) and bathing (0.79), and between the newspaper item and use of objects (0.76). High correlation was also found between contact with others and groupwork (0.77).

Table 4.2: Construct validity: inter-item correlation of the PAL Checklist

	Getting dressed	Eating	Contact with others	Groupwork skills	Communication skills	Practical activities	Use of objects	Looking at a newspaper
Bathing	0.76	0.59	0.65	0.65	0.72	0.79	0.71	0.70
Dressing		0.63	0.63	0.76	0.71	0.80	0.79	0.63
Eating			0.56	0.53	0.75	0.65	0.69	0.60
Contact				0.77	0.72	0.56	0.64	0.68

						0.68	0.69	0.67	0.70
Groupwork						0.68	0.69	0.67	0.70
Communication							0.75	0.80	0.74
Practical								0.81	0.74
Use of objects									0.76

Note: Spearman's rho correlation used

Internal consistency

The Cronbach's alpha coefficient value was 0.95. This statistical test measures the average correlation of all the test items. A minimum value of 0.7 is recommended, and the nearer the value is to 1.0, then the stronger the reliability. This therefore indicates that the scale had excellent internal consistency.

Inter-rater and test–retest reliability

Reliability was measured using two statistical tests: Cohen's kappa and the intraclass coefficient (ICC). Initially, the maximum range of all four activity levels was analysed using a 4 x 4 table. However, because the full range of levels was not used for one item (eating), the ICC values could not be calculated. The data was therefore recoded and analysed, by combining the planned and exploratory activity level results together, and combining the sensory and reflex activity level results together. This reflected the natural division observed within the data, as well as clinical experience of using the PAL Checklist. The kappa and ICC values for inter-rater and test–retest reliability are summarized in Table 4.3. Various 'yardsticks' can be used to define these values, but the following is commonly used: a kappa value of less than 0.40 indicates poor agreement; 0.40 to 0.59 is fair; 0.60 to 0.74 is good; and 0.75 to 1.00 indicates excellent agreement; and an ICC of 0.80 and above indicates that the scale is highly reliable (Bowling 2002). Using these values, all items achieved fair, good or excellent inter-rater and test–retest reliability.

Table 4.3: Reliability: kappa and intraclass coefficient values

	Inter-rater kappa	ICC	Test-rater kappa	ICC
PAL level	0.54	0.69	0.76	0.87
Bathing/washing	0.53	0.61	0.70	0.81
Getting dressed	0.56	0.77	0.76	0.84
Eating	0.94	0.93	1.0	0.96
Contact with others	0.46	0.62	0.57	0.77
Groupwork skills	0.42	0.62	0.58	0.78
Communication skills	0.63	0.72	0.76	0.84
Practical activities	0.66	0.70	0.75	0.86
Use of objects	0.43	0.63	0.55	0.72
Looking at a newspaper	0.57	0.62	0.65	0.75

Note: kappa values: > 0.39 = poor; 0.40 to 0.59 = fair; 0.60 to 0.74 = good; < 0.75 = excellent
Source: Bowling 2002

DISCUSSION

This study showed that the PAL Checklist has adequate validity and reliability and, as such, provides a robust psychometric underpinning for its widespread use in clinical practice. It also suggests that it will also be useful in research with people who have dementia. The questionnaire response rate was excellent. This could be said to indicate the respondents' level of interest in establishing validated tools for use in this setting. The instructions for completion were rated as clear and the checklist was seen as reasonably easy to complete. This reflects the previous anecdotal feedback from practitioners. It would therefore appear to fulfil the original design remit, which was to produce a practical resource for care staff working with people with dementia to enable their engagement in meaningful activities.

Content validity was strong, with most respondents stating that no important items were missing. There was no consistent pattern of response from those suggesting additional items for inclusion. Mood and motivation was suggested as an additional item, but while this is obviously an important factor in selecting and presenting activity, it would not be appropriate to include in a scale that assesses cognitive ability to engage in activity. Another suggestion was the inclusion of orientation and ability to navigate the environment. However, while this depends in part on cognitive components, it is also greatly influenced by the environment itself and how familiar and well designed it is. Lastly, the suggestion to include further daily living activities perhaps reflects the common emphasis on personal care rather than other activities and the tendency observed in some practice settings to use the PAL Checklist as an assessment of daily living activities, which it is not designed to be.

The comments regarding redundant items reflects the first author's clinical experience that care staff in continuing care settings often find the groupwork skills difficult to assess; and that staff in all three settings frequently find the newspaper item difficult to assess as newspapers and magazines are not always routinely available. These comments were also reflected in the ranking of the importance of each item, with the newspaper and groupwork items being scored as very important or essential by 32 per cent and 60 per cent of the respondents respectively. This is a much lower percentage than that given to the other seven items, which were rated at the higher level of importance by more than three-quarters of the respondents.

The frequency of the PAL activity levels and responses for each of the Checklist items within each of the service settings mainly confirmed clinical experience and expectations. However, the absence of anyone being assessed at the sensory activity level within the continuing care settings was surprising and contrasts with the clinical experience of the first author, a specialist practitioner within this area. Perhaps it reflects the difficulty experienced by care staff in differentiating between the PAL activity levels when dealing with people who have more severe dementia, and indeed the tendency to underestimate a person's ability to engage. If so, it appears to reinforce Perrin's (1997, p.938) assertion that 'marked occupational poverty exists' for people with severe dementia.

The results for criterion validity were as predicted, with those people still living in the community achieving higher PAL activity levels. This reflects the relative levels of support and assistance (physical and/or verbal) that people with dementia in different care settings require to carry out activities. In practice, this information can be used to inform and thereby enable caregivers to provide the appropriate level of support to the person, thus moving towards a more optimal balance between providing necessary assistance while also maintaining the individual's remaining abilities and level of independence.

Concurrent validity was high, demonstrating the relevance of taking the level of cognition and severity of dementia into consideration when selecting activities. The importance of using personal history information in combination with the checklist results was highlighted by several respondents. This enables personally meaningful activities to be selected and then presented at the individual's level of ability.

Construct validity was also strong, with the predicted correlation of bathing, dressing, practical activities, use of objects and looking at a newspaper being proven. The strongest correlations were observed between practical activities and the other items, save for the newspaper item, and as such this bears out the clinical expectations. The absence of the newspaper item perhaps reflects the earlier comments reported under content validity. The high correlation between the newspaper item and use of objects supports Pool's original rationale when developing the tool, which included the newspaper item as a way of double checking the ability to handle objects (Pool 2005). The other high correlation between contact with others and groupwork was also anticipated.

The overall reliability of the PAL Checklist was acceptable. The Cronbach's alpha coefficient value indicated excellent internal consistency. This highlights the contribution of each of the items when assessing the ability to engage in activity. Inter-rater reliability was assessed as being fair, with individual items ranging from excellent to fair. The range of values for individual test items perhaps reflects variations in the role of the assessor and the particular service setting. For example, the staff in a day hospital who did not routinely provide personal care assistance found it difficult to assess the bathing and dressing items. Staff were interviewed separately and asked not to confer. This reduced the risk of bias and thereby provided a more rigorous test of reliability. Bearing in mind the number of staff involved in the study, and their differing levels of qualification and experience, the fact that inter-rater reliability for each item was at least fair reflects how quick and easy it is to learn and put into practice with reasonable consistency. Test–retest reliability was assessed as being excellent. This would be expected for a tool that needs to be completed by caregivers who know the person well, measuring a level of performance that would not be expected to change significantly over the course of a week or so. It may therefore be concluded that the PAL Checklist tool demonstrates adequate validity and reliability when used with older people with dementia, and it is also brief, clear and easy to use, and as such can be described as being fit for purpose.

REFERENCES

American Psychiatric Association (1994) *Diagnosis and Statistical Manual of Mental Disorders* (fourth edition). Washington, DC: American Psychiatric Association.

Berg, L., Miller, J.P. and Storandt, M. (1988) 'Mild service dementia of the Alzheimer type: 2. Longitudinal assessment.' *Annals of Neurology*, 23(5), 477–484.

Bowling, A. (2002) *Research Methods in Health: Investigating Health and Health Services* (second edition). Maidenhead: Open University.

Bucks, R.S., Ashworth, D.L., Wilcock, G.K. and Siegfried, K. (1996) 'Development of the Bristol Activities of Daily Living Scale.' *Age and Ageing*, 25(2), 113–120.

Folstein, M.F., Folstein, S.E. and McHugh, P.R. (1975) 'Mini Mental State: A practical guide for grading the cognitive state of patients for the clinician.' *Journal of Psychiatric Research*, 12(3), 189–193.

Hughes, C.P., Berg, L., Danziger, W.L., Coben, L.A. and Martin, R.L. (1982) 'A clinical scale for the staging of dementia.' *British Journal of Psychiatry*, 140, 566–572.

Mahoney, F.I. and Barthel, D.W. (1965) 'Functional evaluation: The Barthel Index.' *Maryland State Medical Journal*, 14, 61–65.

National Institute for Clinical Excellence (NICE) (2006) *Dementia: Supporting People with Dementia and their Carers in Health and Social Care.* National Clinical Practice Guideline number 42. London: NICE.

Pattie, A.H. and Gilleard, C.J. (1979) *Manual of the Clifton Assessment Procedures for the Elderly (CAPE).* Sevenoaks: Hodder and Stoughton Educational.

Perrin, T. (1997) 'Occupational need in severe dementia: A descriptive study.' *Journal of Advanced Nursing*, 25(5), 934–941.

Pool, J. (2002) *The Pool Activity Level (PAL) Instrument for Occupational Profiling* (second edition). London: Jessica Kingsley Publishers.

Pool, J. (2005) Personal communication.

Tombaugh, T.N. and McIntyre, N.J. (1992) 'The Mini-Mental State Examination: A comprehensive review.' *Journal of the American Geriatrics Society*, 40(9), 922–935.

Wade, D.T. and Collin, C. (1988) 'The Barthel ADL Index: A standard measure of physical disability?' *International Disability Studies*, 10, 64–67.

ACKNOWLEDGEMENTS

JW would like to thank all the older people and her colleagues within North East London Mental Health NHS Trust (NELMHT) who contributed to this study, in particular her two co-raters: Jane Burgess and Nicola Elliott, advanced practitioner occupational therapists. She would also like to acknowledge: the funding of her post by the NELMHT Occupational Therapy Service; continued support of the NELMHT Research and Development Directorate; and the College of Occupational Therapists and the Hospital Savings Association for the 2005 PhD Scholarship Award.

This chapter is based on a paper which was originally published as: Wenborn, J., Challis, D., Pool, J., Burgess, J., Elliott, N. and Orrell, M. (2007) 'Assessing the validity and reliability of the Pool Activity Level (PAL) checklist for use with older people with dementia.' We are grateful to the publisher of *Aging and Mental Health*, Taylor and Francis, Abingdon, UK, for permission to reprint some of the content here, with the appropriate contextual alterations.

Chapter 5

VALIDITY AND USE OF THE QCS PAL ENGAGEMENT MEASURE

Lesley Collier and Jackie Pool

To review the utility of and to undertake a basic level of standardization of the Engagement Measure, a number of activities were undertaken involving occupational therapists and people with dementia. Approval from relevant university ethics committees was sought alongside consent for collaboration from health and care settings.

AIM

Overall aim: To assess the reliability, acceptability and validity of the Engagement Measure component of the QCS PAL Instrument for use in hospital and care home settings in order to enhance engagement in activity and well-being of people with dementia.

- To convene a focus group of occupational therapists to identify areas of concern that may be incorporated into the Engagement Measure.
- To design and pilot the Engagement Measure.
- To gather qualitative feedback from therapists using the Engagement Measure.
- To undertake quantitative analysis of the Engagement Measure during engagement in activity.

BACKGROUND

Engaging in meaningful activity is a key component of an active lifestyle, maintaining autonomy, well-being and self-esteem as we age (Kim *et al.* 2012; Leone *et al.* 2012). Paradoxically, a diagnosis of dementia will often trigger a reduction in engagement in activity, which in turn leads to increased levels of dependency (Chung 2004; Morgan-Brown, Newton and Ormerod 2012). This disruption in activity is often reflected in the person's actions, with searching behaviour that may reflect boredom, while aggression and agitation may indicate frustration at not being able to take part in activity (Collier *et al.* 2010; Gori, Pientini and Vespa 2001). Government initiatives such as the Prime Minister's Challenge on Dementia (Department of Health 2020) have endeavoured to tackle the problem of engaging people with dementia in activity, and *Care Management for Older People with Serious Mental Health Problems* (Department of Health 2002) also endeavours to address the challenges presented by people with dementia. The key to improved care is the use of standardized assessment, and the PAL Instrument for Occupational Profiling addresses this, particularly as it is a bespoke system for use with people with dementia and its main focus is on engagement in activity and therapeutic environments. By extending its use to include an outcome measure, formal and informal carers will be able to identify whether the PAL programme of activity has been structured to maximize opportunities for increasing engagement in personal and meaningful activities.

This study aimed to standardize the Engagement Measure that was designed to be used in parallel with the PAL Occupational Profiling Tool. The Engagement Measure has the potential to measure such changes which are known to be associated with improved functioning in activities of daily living and reduction in carer burden (Graff *et al.* 2006).

BENEFIT TO INDIVIDUALS WITH COGNITIVE IMPAIRMENT

This study addressed a core feature identified as influencing well-being and engagement in people with dementia by both the person themselves and those who care for them. Initial work undertaken by Wenborn *et al.* (2008) using the PAL suggested that activity could be structured to be accessible for people with mild through to severe dementia. Early feedback from carers reported that this tool allowed them to interact successfully with the person with dementia, increased sense of well-being and reduced incidences of distressed behaviours and perceptions of burden. This may be explained by several features that are known to be influenced by activity (Crombie *et al.* 2004). Activity being of the suitable level and of interest to the participant is an important feature to ensure success (Leone *et al.* 2012). Having a purpose and opportunity to engage in activity is also considered to have a direct correlation with well-being and a sense of identity (Fung, Leung and Lam 2011; Lu and Haase 2011). Although the PAL helps to structure activity at an appropriate level, having a standardized system to measure whether these features have been addressed will increase well-being and autonomy in older people with dementia, which will also have a direct impact on perceived carer burden. In care management, achieving well-being for the person with dementia is a key deliverable of the Care Quality Commission (CQC), along with achieving job satisfaction for the health and social care professional and monitoring performance outcomes. Involving people with dementia in the development of this Engagement Measure ensured that it has a good face validity and measures aspects that are important. As it is also anticipated that carers will use the PAL and the new Engagement Measure, involving carers in the design ensured that appropriate languages are used and the user interface is accessible. It is envisaged that the new Engagement Measure will be used alongside the PAL to further explore the efficacy of activity engagement for people with dementia and to explore ways of reducing the perceived caring burden for those people who are cared for at home, in care homes and also in the hospital environment.

EXPERTS BY EXPERIENCE INVOLVEMENT

During the initial development of this proposal a number of people with dementia and their families were approached to ask about how this Engagement Measure may help them manage their everyday life. Families often reported they found it difficult to choose appropriate activities and were not sure if they had got it right when they tried. They agreed that having an easy tool to help them would be of benefit and especially so when the person with dementia had to move to a care home as it would help care staff 'understand them better'.

There was further significant involvement in this study of both people with dementia and their carers (family, friends and informal carers) within the formal structure of the study. People with dementia and their carers were involved in the analysis phase. As the PAL Instrument was designed to be accessible to informal carers as well as paid care staff, the language used in the Engagement Measure needed also to be appropriate. During the analysis phase, people with dementia in a care home setting participated in activities and were assessed using the Engagement Measure. As such, their comments on the Engagement Measure were recorded.

PLAN OF INVESTIGATION

Study design

This study used a combination of a qualitative focus-group-driven phase followed by a pilot quantitative study to determine validity of the Engagement Measure to be used in partnership with the PAL Instrument for Occupational Profiling.

Selection of participants

Focus group phase – this phase involved occupational therapy staff within the South East region of the UK. Participants were recruited following an introductory meeting with one of the research team. Those who were interested in joining the focus group were given an information sheet and details of how to register their interest with the research team. Following recruitment, a date was organized for the focus groups to take place.

Analysis phase – participants in this phase were residents in a care home setting who met the DSM-IV-TR (American Psychiatric Association 2000) diagnostic criteria for dementia and scored less than 24 on the Montreal Cognitive Assessment (MoCA) (Nasreddine *et al.* 2005). Consent was gained using guidelines from the Mental Capacity Act (2005).

Exclusion – participants for the focus group phase were excluded if they did not work with people with dementia and/or had limited understanding of written English. Participants for the analysis phase were excluded if they became too unwell to participate in activity or were discharged from the care setting.

Sample size and justification

A convenience sample was used based on available access to several care settings using the PAL Instrument within the South East region. It was estimated that 30 participants would be recruited for the analysis phase based on current contact figures within community settings within the proposed region.

ETHICAL CONSIDERATIONS

The University of Southampton Ethics Committee was approached for approval. Consent for those volunteering to take part in the focus groups was sought via formal written consent prior to the start of the group. For the analysis phase, given the relative severity of cognitive impairment in the participants, individuals as well as their principal carers were approached for formal consent. Where the individual was unable to understand or retain relevant information regarding the study, verbal assent was sought from the principal caregiver. In this case, ongoing consent from the participant was ascertained via non-verbal behaviour. As far as was possible, explanation was given to every participant about the interventions they were taking part in. All participants were free to withdraw from the study at any point. In addition, careful attention was paid to their non-verbal communication, so if the participant appeared to find any part of the study distressing, they were withdrawn. The members of the research team who were involved in gathering data from participants in care homes had considerable experience in working and engaging with people with dementia.

PROCEDURE

Focus group phase – a focus group with occupational therapy staff was held to discuss the content of the Engagement Measure and areas of importance that should be included. The focus group was facilitated by a member of the research team. Feedback was recorded by a scribe. The focus group comments formed consensus on:

- operational definitions of the components of the Engagement Measure developed from the original item pool
- priority and relevance of components (are components redundant and are important components missing?)
- clarity of instructions regarding the use and content of the Engagement Measure.

Once amended, this second version of the Engagement Measure was piloted in a care home setting.

Analysis phase – the pilot phase was undertaken in a care home setting where the PAL Instrument was currently used. Participants were older people with dementia. A member of staff from the care home setting completed the MoCA (Nasreddine *et al.* 2005) and the PAL Checklist of function to determine level of function and of occupational performance, against which the Engagement Measure was evaluated. The member of staff working with the participant also kept a diary of reported observations of how the participant's engagement in activity had changed over the past two weeks. Any comments regarding the Engagement Measure given by the participant and their carers were also recorded.

A summary of the procedure is illustrated in Table 5.1.

Table 5.1: Summary of the procedure

Phase 1 Focus groups	Phase 2 Analysis	Consolidation – two weeks
Focus groups to assist in the construction of the Engagement Measure	Completion of MoCA, PAL Checklist of function, PAL Engagement Measure	Completion of activity programme
Circulation of version 1 to users of PAL Instrument	Construction of activity programme	Ongoing engagement diary
Initial pilot and adaptation of version 2		Use of version 2 Engagement Measure

RESULTS: FOCUS GROUP

The group comprised of five occupational therapists with experience of using the PAL with older people with dementia. The group discussion was recorded with permission, transcribed, and analysed using thematic analysis (Braun and Clarke 2006).

Some key themes emerged.

'It feels user friendly'

This theme related to the accessibility and utility of the Engagement Measure. Participants noted that the terminology felt familiar, and it helped to see the progression of an individual over time. Suggestions for improvement included colour coordinating the sections to help with orientation to the form.

'Technology is familiar and comfortable...'

'I use the electronic option to fill colour in the cells.'

'Additional categories'

This theme related to the sub-categories in the Engagement Measure. Participants felt the sub-categories were appropriate and the definitions given. Comments were given regarding the ordering of the sub-categories and the relevance to activity description.

'Possibly it would flow better if it was in the order that a person engages in physical components.'

'It [sub-categories] fits well with the PAL.'

'Demonstrating the value of what we are doing'

This theme reflected participants' beliefs of what the Engagement Measure achieved. There was a recognition that the measure provided evidence to demonstrate the value of what they were doing. The results had impact on service delivery and influenced positively perceptions of other healthcare professionals in occupational therapy. Participants felt the Engagement Measure illustrated the benefits of participating in activities for individuals with dementia, and the achievements made regardless of the time spent in the activity.

'We can see the impact we are having...'

'Some staff are saying a patient didn't like the music group because they didn't stay very long, but we are able to show that she did gain a lot even though she was only able to engage a short while.'

'Feedback from psychology colleagues...we are doing something more complex than they had realized.'

'I like the term engagement measure'

This theme summarized the overall perspective of the measure. Participants felt it was useful and one of the few tools available to measure engagement. They also felt it helped with goal setting, with the ability to focus on specific activity.

'It helps with measuring outcome from admission to discharge...'

'I like the term engagement measure because it is what we are measuring.'

'It's really whetted my appetite; I want to use it more and get more out of it.'

RECOMMENDATIONS

A number of recommendations were identified from the focus group and included in the second version of the Engagement Measure.

1. Colour coordination of sub-categories to help with orientation to the Engagement Measure.
2. Ordering of the sub-categories to more accurately reflect the engagement in activity process.
3. Further description of how to use the measure to ensure it is accessible to other health and social care professionals.

RESULTS: ANALYSIS

Descriptive statistics

Participants were recruited from a care home in the South East. Demographics of the participant group are illustrated in Table 5.2.

Table 5.2: Demographics of participants

n = 13	Range	Mean	Standard deviation
Age	77–95 years	89 years	6 years

n = 13	Male	Female
Gender	5	8

Participants were assessed at baseline using the Neurobehavioural Rating Scale (NRS) (Sultzer *et al.* 1992), the QCS PAL Instrument for Occupational Profiling (Pool 2012), and the QCS Pool Activity Engagement Measure. Baseline data are recorded in Tables 5.3, 5.4 and 5.5.

Table 5.3: PAL baseline scores

PAL criteria	Planned	Exploratory	Sensory	Reflex
Number of participants	3	6	3	1

Table 5.4: NRS baseline scores

NRS criteria	Mean	Standard deviation	Skewness
NRS-A (Cognition/Insight)	18	8.78	.54
NRS-B (Agitation/Disinhibition)	8.54	9.19	1.77
NRS-C (Behavioural retardation)	2.38	2.84	1.87

NRS-D (Anxiety/Depression)	2.54	4.96	2.90
NRS-E (Verbal output)	.92	1.18	1.58
NRS-F (Psychosis)	2.31	4.27	1.99

Table 5.5: PAL Engagement Measure baseline scores (PALEM) criteria

	Mean	Standard deviation	Skewness
PALEM Cognitive ability	15.08	4.42	−.14
PALEM Social interaction	8.38	2.50	.01
PALEM Physical ability	11.46	3.20	−.21
PALEM Emotional well-being	7.85	2.99	.08

Tests were undertaken to explore whether baseline data improved in terms of mood, behaviour and engagement. The PAL engagement scores improved over time (t (3) = 14.03, p = .001), suggesting there was an improvement in engagement scores. In particular, cognitive abilities including goal awareness, initiation, attention, concentration, exploration and response improved. Additionally, physical ability including coordination, manipulation and handling of objects improved. Scores for the NRS did not change significantly except for cognitive/insight, which included relating to others, increased speed of movement and increased emotional tone and intensity of emotional response (t (3) = 5.51, p = .012).

CONCLUSION

The outcome of this study revealed that the utility of the Engagement Measure was perceived as good by occupational therapists using the measure. They felt it accurately described engagement in terms of the sub-categories and was easy to use. They suggested that the layout be adjusted to reflect the process of engagement and the form be colour coordinated to assist with orientation and scoring.

The qualitative element revealed that the Engagement Measure was sensitive to change and illustrated an improvement in engagement that was aligned with improvement in behaviour, including relating to others, dexterity and emotional interaction. Further analysis should be undertaken to further determine sensitivity to change and content validity.

EXAMPLE OF THE QCS PAL ENGAGEMENT MEASURE USED IN PRACTICE

The following case study provides an example of how the PAL Engagement Measure can be used to record the way that an individual has engaged in a specific activity over a time period. This can help to identify aspects to focus on in order to support the individual to improve or maintain their functional ability. The PAL Engagement Measure can also be used as part of a reflective practice supervision of care or activity team members as it identifies how the individual has been supported to engage in a specific activity and can illustrate how the team member has improved their support. It can also be used as an outcome measure for evidencing the usefulness of a new activity resource that might be being trialled in a care setting.

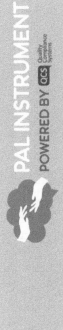

QCS PAL ENGAGEMENT MEASURE

PAL INSTRUMENT
POWERED BY QCS

Guidance for use:

1. Complete this sheet for up to 4 sessions of the same activity that the person is participating in
2. Decide the frequency of your observed recording (daily, weekly, monthly)
3. Enter the date of the observed activity in the date cell
4. Score 0,1 or 2 as indicated on the score sheet in the column
5. The cell will automatically highlight red, yellow or green to correspond with the numerical score as indicated
6. Compare across columns to evaluate the impact of the activity, either by score and/or colour code
7. The Engagement Measure colours will graphically illustrate how the person has engaged and their changes over time

You can choose the frequency that you complete this measure. It will support you to provide evidence of an indidividual's participation in everyday life to family members or to inspectors and regulators. It can also help to objectively identify the level of service the person needs. You could also use the measure to monitor the impact of your activity provision

NAME: James Brown	Measure 1	Measure 2	Measure 3	Measure 4	NOT OBSERVED DURING THE ACTIVITY (0 Point)	OBSERVED AT TIMES (1 Point)	OBSERVED CONSISTENTLY (2 Points)
OBSERVED ACTIVITY: Dining							
Date:	6/1/2022	6/8/2022	6/15/2022	6/22/2022			
COGNITIVE ABILITIES							
Goal aware	1	1	1	2	Has an end result in mind, can plan how to achieve and work towards this		
Initiates	1	1	1	1	Independently starts an action toward another person or object		
Attends	0	1	1	2	Notices and focuses on a sensation		
Concentrates	1	1	1	1	Sustains attention on the activity, person or object		
Adjusts	2	2	2	2	Adapts actions to meet the demands of the activity		
Explores	0	1	1	2	Shows interest in and seeks to engage with environment, people or objects		
Responds	0	0	1	2	Reacts to sensations, verbal requests or prompts		

PHYSICAL ABILITIES				
Stabilizes	0	1	2	Maintains balance and posture while moving, standing or sitting
Manipulates	2	2	2	Uses tools and objects to achieve an end result. Handles an object in response to the sensation it generates
Coordinates	0	1	1	Moves smoothly while negotiating obstacles of handling objects
Grips objects	2	2	2	Uses appropriate strength to hold objects securely
Releases objects	1	2	2	Independently and appropriately lets go of objects
SOCIAL INTERACTION				
Aware of others	1	2	2	Notices and responds directly or indirectly to the presence of others
Shares	0	1	2	Offers and accepts objects to/from others
Vocal interactions	2	2	2	Uses vocal sounds to make a connection with others
Non-vocal interactions	2	2	2	Uses body language to make a connection with others
EMOTIONAL WELL-BEING				
Hope	0	1	2	Shows a sense of optimism in engaging in the activity
Agency	1	1	2	Shows a sense of purposefulness in carrying out the activity
Self-confidence	0	1	2	Shows a sense of empowerment and autonomy when carrying out the activity
Self-esteem	1	1	1	Shows a sense of fulfilment when carrying out and on completion of the activity
% Engagement Achieved	43	58	73	90

PLEASE REMEMBER TO SAVE YOUR WORKSHEET EACH TIME YOU COMPLETE IT

Figure 5.1: Completed example of the QCS PAL Engagement Measure

JAMES BROWN

James has recently moved into Primrose Care Home and the team is concerned about his well-being as he does not eat well and is losing weight. James has a diagnosis of Lewy body disease and has symptoms that include a hand tremor, rigid facial muscles, difficulty making sense of what he sees as well as difficulty with sitting upright. He is slowed in his ability to process conversations and to respond and he seems reluctant to join other residents at the dining table, not taking part in conversations or responding to requests, such as to pass the salt or to share the water jug.

The dining room team is keen to support James to have a better dining experience and feels that, if his abilities are improved or his difficulties compensated for, he will have more confidence in dining with others and will eat better as well.

They complete the PAL Engagement Measure to find out what aspects James is specifically struggling with and to address those that will help him. The team also completes the PAL Checklist and identifies that James is currently at an exploratory level of ability, although his Lewy body symptoms and his low self-esteem are undermining his ability to show interest in and seek to engage with the dining room environment and other residents.

As James is having difficulty with using cutlery because of his hand tremor and in sitting upright at the dining table, the team manager refers to the Community Mental Health Team for Older People for an occupational therapist to assess his needs and provide support. Meanwhile, the team provides him with some weighted cutlery and uses cushions for sitting support. When the occupational therapist assesses, a specific chair is recommended that provides good stability for James to sit well at the dining table.

As James is not attending to the visual sensations of dining, the team tries offering his food on a red plate so that there is a good colour contrast. This works well, and to add to this, the team plans to always describe to him what is on his plate as they serve him and to also encourage him to enjoy the smell of the food. They see his ability to attend improve quickly because of this approach.

In addition, the team member who is supporting the dining on James's table stimulates social discussion and supports the conversation to be slowed to a pace that James can more easily follow, allowing time for him to respond.

James becomes more self-confident in his abilities at the dining table, eats better and his weight improves. The PAL Engagement Measure evidences his improvements, which is great for team morale and also for his daughters, who are delighted to see this clear dedication to supporting their dad's unique needs. A further PAL Checklist is completed which identifies that James is now at a planned level of ability.

REFERENCES

American Psychiatric Association (2000) *Diagnostic and Statistical Manual of Mental Disorders* (fourth edition text revision). Washington, DC: American Psychiatric Association.

Braun, V. and Clarke, V. (2006) 'Using thematic analysis in psychology.' *Qualitative Research in Psychology*, 3(2), 77–101, doi: 10.1191/1478088706qp063oa.

Chung, J. (2004) 'Activity participation and well-being of people with dementia in long-term care settings.' *OTJR-Occupation, Participation and Health*, 24, 22–31.

Collier, L., McPherson, K., Ellis-Hill, C., Staal, J. and Bucks, R. (2010) 'Multisensory stimulation to improve functional performance in moderate to severe dementia – Interim results.' *American Journal of Alzheimer's Disease and Other Dementias*, 25(8), 698–703.

Crombie, I., Irvine, L., Williams, B., McGinnis, A. *et al.* (2004) 'Why older people do not participate in leisure time physical activity: A survey of activity levels, beliefs and deterrents.' *Age and Ageing*, 33(3), 287–292.

Department of Health (2002) *Care Management for Older People with Serious Mental Health Problems.* London: Department of Health.

Department of Health (2020) *The Prime Minister's Challenge on Dementia.* London: Department of Health.

Fung, A.W., Leung, G.T. and Lam, L.C. (2011) 'Modulating factors that preserve cognitive function in healthy ageing.' *East Asian Archives of Psychiatry*, 21(4), 152–156.

Gori, G., Pientini, S. and Vespa, A. (2001) 'The selection of meaningful activities as a treatment for day-care in dementia.' *Archives of Gerontology and Geriatrics*, Supplement 7, 207–212.

Graff, M., Vernooij-Dassen, M., Thijssen, M., Dekker, J., Hoefnagels, W. and Olde Rikkert, M. (2006) 'Community occupational therapy for older patients with dementia and their care givers: Randomised controlled trial.' *British Medical Journal*, 333, 1196–1202.

Kim, S.Y., Yoo, E.Y., Jung, M.Y., Park, S.H. and Park, J.H. (2012) 'A systematic review of the effects of occupational therapy for persons with dementia: A meta-analysis of randomized controlled trials.' *Neurorehabilitation*, 31(2), 107–115.

Leone, E., Piano, J., Deudon, A., Alain, B. *et al.* (2012) 'What are you interested in? A survey on 601 nursing homes residents activities interests.' *Advances in Aging Research*, 1(2), 13–21.

Lu, Y.Y. and Haase, J.E. (2011) 'Content validity and acceptability of the daily enhancement of meaningful activity program: Intervention for mild cognitive impairment patient-spouse dyads.' *Journal of Neuroscience Nursing*, 43(6), 317–328.

Mental Capacity Act (2005) London: The Stationery Office.

Morgan-Brown, M., Newton, R. and Ormerod, M. (2012) 'Engaging life in two Irish nursing home units for people with dementia: Quantitative comparisons before and after implementing household environments.' *Aging and Mental Health*, 3 Sept [Epub ahead of print].

Nasreddine, Z.S., Phillips, N.A., Bédirian, V., Charbonneau, S. *et al.* (2005) 'The Montreal Cognitive Assessment (MoCA): A brief screening tool for mild cognitive impairment.' *Journal of the American Geriatrics Society*, 53, 695–699.

Pool, J. (2012) *The Pool Activity Level (PAL) Instrument for Occupational Profiling: A Practical Resource for Carers of People with Cognitive Impairment.* 4th ed. University of Bradford Dementia Good Practice Guides. London: Jessica Kingsley Publishers.

Sultzer, D.L., Levin, H.S., Mahler, M.E., High, W.M. and Cummings, J.L. (1992) 'Assessment of cognitive, psychiatric, and behavioral disturbances in patients with dementia: The Neurobehavioral Rating Scale.' *Journal of the American Geriatrics Society*, 40(6), 549–555.

Wenborn, J., Challis, D., Pool, J., Burgess, J., Elliott, N. and Orrell, M. (2008) Assessing the validity and reliability of the Pool Activity Level (PAL) checklist for use with older people with dementia. *Aging and Mental Health*, 12, 202–211.

Chapter 6

LIFE HISTORY WORK

THE IMPORTANCE OF GATHERING A LIFE HISTORY

Life history or story work is recognized as an important process that is a major influence in care planning as a means of 'engaging and interacting with people of different ages in order to encourage and assist them to recall and to record in tangible form their personal histories' (Gibson 2005, pp.175–179). Wray (2021, pp.81–82) described how our identity is created from our lived experiences and, as people's dementia progresses, their struggle to bring the details of their life back to mind can deplete their sense of identity. Providing people living with a dementia with the opportunity to express their character and personality, to engage in familiar routines and habits and to re-experience the sensory and functional use of objects supports them to reconnect with their identity and sense of self. Enabling this engagement is possible for people at all levels of dementia.

Life history differs from life review in that it does not require an evaluation of the information that is gathered. Whereas life review is a therapeutic approach to resolving past problems, life history work is not directly aimed at changing the view of himself or herself held by the person, but rather at caregivers who are encouraged to recognize the whole person in the context of their lifespan. The factual account of an individual's life history builds up a full picture of the person. This perspective should assist caregivers in their interactions with the person and in planning activities that relate to the person's interests and experiences. The result of this individualized care plan is to recognize the uniqueness of the person and to potentially make a significant change in the quality of their life. The purpose of a Personal History Profile is to enable carers to recognize the person as a unique individual and not only to see the person's disability.

The PAL Instrument Personal History Profile is a method that uses subheadings to guide the user when gathering relevant information. By finding out about all that the person has experienced it is possible to have a better understanding of the person's behaviour now. It also gives care workers, who may not know the person very well, topics of conversation that will have meaning for the person.

Putting together the Profile should be an enjoyable project that the person with cognitive impairment, relatives and care workers can join together in, encouraging social interaction and reminiscence. The information gained from the Personal History Profile informs the PAL Activity Profile by guiding activity selection.

GUIDELINES FOR GATHERING LIFE HISTORY INFORMATION USING THE PAL PERSONAL HISTORY PROFILE

The questions in the Profile are very general, designed to cater for all people regardless of age or sex. Some questions may be irrelevant, and these should be ignored. If the person is being cared for in a care home or hospital or is attending a day centre, it may be possible to ask family members to complete the whole form with the person at home. For others, completion of the Profile may be spread out over a period of weeks, as more information is revealed. The Profile is therefore not an assessment but a means of recording useful information in a systematic way.

Any photographs that are available can be added to the Profile. It is helpful to write on the reverse the person's name, who is in the photograph and where and when it was taken. Some relatives may be worried about the photographs getting lost or damaged. In these cases, the photographs can be photocopied, and the originals kept safe.

A sample of a completed Profile is included for information.

REFERENCES

Gibson, F. (2005) 'Fit for Life: The Contribution of Life Story Work.' In M. Marshall (ed.) *Perspectives on Rehabilitation and Dementia*. London: Jessica Kingsley Publishers.

Wray, A. (2021) *Why Dementia Makes Communication Difficult*. London: Jessica Kingsley Publishers.

POOL ACTIVITY LEVEL (PAL) PERSONAL HISTORY PROFILE

What is your name? *Elsie Jones*

When were you born? *10 November 1936*

CHILDHOOD
Where were you born?
Leeds, West Riding of Yorkshire

What are your family members' names?
Thomas and Molly Charlton (parents), Harry (older brother)

What were your family members' occupations?
Sweet shop owners (parents)
Tram driver (brother, Harry) but died in 1966

Where did you live?
Headingley, Leeds

Which schools did you attend?
Leeds Girls' School

What was your favourite subject?
English and Sewing

Did you have any family pets? What were their names?
Cats: Charlie and Smudge

ADOLESCENCE
When did you leave school?
Age 15

Where did you work?
Parents' shop, then went to clothing factory, then opened own shop in York in 1962

What did you do at work?
Machinist at factory, then owned dress shop

Did you have any special training?
Can't remember

What special memories do you have of work days?
Day trips in summer. Friend, Mary, machined across her finger

✓

ADULTHOOD

Do/did you have a partner? What is your partner's name and occupation?
Sidney, bank clerk

Where and when did you meet?
At a dance in Leeds

Where and when did you marry?
5 May 1956 at Headingley Church

Where did you go on your honeymoon?
Scarborough

Where did you live?
Leeds, moved to York when Sidney was promoted

Do you have any children? What are their names?
Shirley, March 1957

Do you have any grandchildren? What are their names?
Susan, 1977, and Michael, 1979

Did you have any special friends? What are their names?
Barbara

When and where did you meet?
Factory

Are you still in touch?
See each other sometimes

Did you have any pets? What were their names?
Cats, latest one Susie is 19 years old

RETIREMENT

When did you retire?
1996 age 60. Sidney retired from bank in 2001

What were you looking forward to most?
Gardening together, touring, visiting family

What were your hobbies and interests?
Used to sew and read a lot but stopped when eyes got bad

What were the biggest changes for you?
Shirley moving away to London when she married

LIKES AND DISLIKES

What do you enjoy doing now?

Like to listen to big band music, and to story tapes. Quizzes on the television

What do you like to read?

Thrillers, Agatha Christie

What is your favourite colour?

Yellow

What kind of music do you like?

Big band, Nat King Cole

What are your favourite foods and drinks?

Soup, sandwiches, sherry

Is there anything that you definitely do not like to do?

Bingo

HOW YOU LIKE TO DO THINGS

Do you have any special routines to your day?

Main meal at lunch time, bath before bed and hot chocolate in bed to settle me

What time do you like to get up in the morning? And go to bed at night?

Get up at 9, go to bed after 10 o'clock news

Do you want people to help you with anything?

Doing up fastenings and getting in and out of the bath

Do you want people to leave you to do anything on your own?

Having a bath, getting dressed, except for fastenings

How do you like people to address you?

Elsie

What are you good at?

Quizzes

Is there anything else you would like to tell us about you?

No

Chapter 7

QCS PAL CHECKLIST CASE STUDIES

The following case studies give examples of how the PAL Checklist can be used to record the way that an individual carries out everyday activities in order to identify their level of cognitive ability.

The first four case studies reveal that each individual is entirely at one level for all activities. The final three are intended to illustrate how a checklist may be completed for individuals who have a range of abilities across the activities.

CASE STUDY 1

John Porter is a retired headteacher who lives with his wife. He is a very precise man who enjoys propagating plants and stamp collecting. Six months ago, John went to his GP because he was worried about his increasingly poor memory. The GP diagnosed Alzheimer's disease. This is affecting John's ability to remember the names of friends, plants and stamps in his collection and he finds this frustrating and embarrassing. His wife is worried that this will lower John's confidence when out and will affect their weekly outings to local restaurants. Although he is able to select cutlery appropriately, he has become less socially outgoing and does not chat to the waiters as he used to.

Although John does have memory problems and is now not paying so much attention to the finer details and finishing touches in his hobbies, he still enjoys being involved in his hobbies with his wife's help.

When John is at ease with others, he is able to start conversations and enjoys discussing topics that he has noticed in the newspaper. Only people close to him realize that he has any disability, and only last week John enjoyed an afternoon with two close friends, when they all successfully constructed and painted a new garden shed. There was one moment when he had difficulty with aligning the hinges on the door and could not solve the problem, but one of the others stepped in to help and John was able to carry on with another part of the project.

John is also able to use his own initiative to carry out most everyday tasks. Although his wife has to remind him to have a wash and to shave, John is able to choose what to wear and to get dressed independently.

John and his wife are keen to plan ways of continuing his independence for as long as possible. When the Pool Activity Level (PAL) Checklist is completed for John it reveals that he is able to carry out activities at a *planned* activity level. It is now possible to use this information to help John to use his remaining abilities and to compensate for his disabilities.

QCS POOL ACTIVITY LEVEL (PAL) CHECKLIST

Name: *John Porter*

Date: *1 September 2022*

Completed by: A care worker

> Activity Level indicated: Planned

Ensure you are familiar with the instructions before completion

Completing the Checklist	Key
• Thinking of the last two weeks, tick the statement that represents the person's ability in each section.	P = Planned level of ability
• If in doubt about which statement to tick, choose the level of ability that represents their average performance over the last two weeks.	E = Exploratory level of ability S = Sensory level of ability
• There should only be ONE TICK for each section.	R = Reflex level of ability
• You must tick one statement for each section.	
• Total the ticks at the bottom of each column over page.	

1. Bathing/Washing	P	E	S	R
• Can bathe/wash independently, sometimes with a little help to start	✓			
• Needs soap put on flannel and one-step-at-a-time directions to wash				
• Mainly relies on others but will wipe own face and hands if encouraged				
• Totally dependent and needs full assistance to wash or bathe				

2. Getting dressed	P	E	S	R
• Plans what to wear, selects own clothing from the cupboards; dresses in correct order	✓			
• Needs help to plan what to wear but recognizes items and how to wear them; needs help with order of dressing				
• Needs help to plan and with order of dressing, but can carry out small activities if someone directs each step				
• Totally dependent on someone to plan, sequence and complete dressing; may move limbs to assist				

3. Eating	P	E	S	R
• Eats independently and using the correct cutlery	✓			
• Eats using a spoon and/or needs food to be cut up into small pieces				
• Only uses fingers to eat food				
• Relies on others to be fed				

4. Contact with others	P	E	S	R
• Initiates social contact and responds to the needs of others	✓			
• Aware of others and will seek interaction, but may be more concerned with own needs				
• Aware of others but waits for others to make the first social contact				
• May not show an awareness of the presence of others unless in direct physical contact				
5. Groupwork skills	**P**	**E**	**S**	**R**
• Engages with others in a group activity, can take turns with the activity/tools	✓			
• Occasionally engages with others in a group, moving in and out of the group at a whim				
• Aware of others in the group and will work alongside others, although tends to focus on own activity				
• Does not show awareness of others in the group unless close one-to-one attention is experienced				
6. Communication skills	**P**	**E**	**S**	**R**
• Is aware of appropriate interaction, can chat coherently and is able to use complex language skills	✓			
• Body language may be inappropriate and may not always be coherent, but can use simple language skills				
• Responses to verbal interaction may be mainly through body language; comprehension is limited				
• Can only respond to direct physical contact from others through touch, eye contact or facial expression				
7. Practical activities (craft, domestic chores, gardening)	**P**	**E**	**S**	**R**
• Can plan to carry out an activity, hold the goal in mind and work through a familiar sequence; may need help solving problems	✓			
• More interested in the making or doing than the end result, needs prompting to remember purpose, can get distracted				
• Activities need to be broken down and presented one step at a time, multisensory stimulation can help hold the attention				
• Unable to 'do' activities, but responds to the close contact of others and experiencing physical sensations				
8. Use of objects	**P**	**E**	**S**	**R**
• Plans to use and looks for objects that are not visible; may struggle if objects are not in usual/familiar places (e.g. toiletries in a bathroom cupboard)	✓			
• Selects objects appropriately only if in view (e.g. toiletries on a shelf next to the washbasin)				
• Randomly uses objects as chances on them; may use appropriately				
• May grip objects when placed in the hand but will not attempt to use them				

9. Looking at a newspaper/magazine	P	E	S	R
• Comprehends and shows interest in the content, turns the pages and looks at headlines and pictures	✓			
• Turns the pages randomly, only attending to items pointed out by others				
• Will hold and may feel the paper, but will not turn the pages unless directed and will not show interest in the content				
• May grip the paper if it is placed in the hand but may not be able to release the grip; or may not take hold of the paper				
NB: If the totals are evenly divided between activity levels, assume that the person is at the lower level but has the potential to move into the higher level. **Totals**	9	0	0	0

The Activity Level identified for this person is: Planned

Transfer this information to the front of the form.

> Now use the relevant PAL Activity Profile to assist you to plan how you will help the person with their activities.

CASE STUDY 2

Elsie Jones is a retired businesswoman who owned her own dress shop. Her family have old photographs showing that Elsie was a very well-groomed woman, but sadly she now struggles to dress herself. Elsie is determined to dress herself, but she often looks dishevelled, with petticoats hanging under the hemline of her dress, or put on top of her dress, and her hair untidy. Elsie shows that she is aware of her appearance and is often seen tugging at her dress to pull it over the petticoat, and smoothing down her hair with her hands.

Elsie has vascular dementia and she lives with her daughter and family. They are asking for advice about how they can help Elsie to look smart again without taking away her independence and doing everything for her. Her daughter explains that Elsie relies on prompts to have a wash, which she can do if the cloth is prepared and passed to her. She is able to eat her meals using a spoon, but struggles to use a knife and fork.

Elsie's family are also concerned that she tries to help with chores but gives up when she cannot find things, and that she tends to blame others, saying someone has not put them away in the right place. For example, Elsie recently became very cross with her granddaughter and accused her of taking her make-up bag, which had actually been tidied away into the top drawer of Elsie's dressing table.

Also, if something else attracts Elsie's attention, she will leave tasks unfinished. This causes a great deal of untidiness in the home. Elsie has always been a very sociable woman and she continues to make superficial conversation with others at the local day centre, which she visits weekly. However, she tends mainly to focus on her own needs and does not respond to the others in her arts and crafts group if they express any distress or discomfort. She enjoys chatting to her grandchildren when the conversation is about simple and familiar events, although she tends to switch off if more complex topics are discussed. Elsie's granddaughter, Susan, likes to sit and look at *Woman and Home* magazine with her, although Elsie tends only to look at articles when Susan points them out.

When the Pool Activity Level (PAL) Checklist is completed for Elsie it reveals that she is able to carry out activities at an *exploratory* activity level. It is now possible to use this information in the Activity Profile to help Elsie to use her remaining abilities and to compensate for her disabilities.

QCS POOL ACTIVITY LEVEL (PAL) CHECKLIST

Name: Elsie Jones

Date: 1 September 2022

Completed by: A care worker

> Activity Level indicated: Exploratory

Ensure you are familiar with the instructions before completion

Completing the Checklist	Key
• Thinking of the last two weeks, tick the statement that represents the person's ability in each section. • If in doubt about which statement to tick, choose the level of ability that represents their average performance over the last two weeks. • There should only be ONE TICK for each section. • You must tick one statement for each section. • Total the ticks at the bottom of each column over page.	P = Planned level of ability E = Exploratory level of ability S = Sensory level of ability R = Reflex level of ability

1. Bathing/Washing	P	E	S	R
• Can bathe/wash independently, sometimes with a little help to start				
• Needs soap put on flannel and one-step-at-a-time directions to wash		✓		
• Mainly relies on others but will wipe own face and hands if encouraged				
• Totally dependent and needs full assistance to wash or bathe				

2. Getting dressed	P	E	S	R
• Plans what to wear, selects own clothing from the cupboards; dresses in correct order				
• Needs help to plan what to wear but recognizes items and how to wear them; needs help with order of dressing		✓		
• Needs help to plan and with order of dressing, but can carry out small activities if someone directs each step				
• Totally dependent on someone to plan, sequence and complete dressing; may move limbs to assist				

3. Eating	P	E	S	R
• Eats independently and using the correct cutlery				
• Eats using a spoon and/or needs food to be cut up into small pieces		✓		
• Only uses fingers to eat food				
• Relies on others to be fed				

4. Contact with others	P	E	S	R
• Initiates social contact and responds to the needs of others				
• Aware of others and will seek interaction, but may be more concerned with own needs		✓		
• Aware of others but waits for others to make the first social contact				
• May not show an awareness of the presence of others unless in direct physical contact				
5. Groupwork skills	P	E	S	R
• Engages with others in a group activity, can take turns with the activity/tools				
• Occasionally engages with others in a group, moving in and out of the group at a whim		✓		
• Aware of others in the group and will work alongside others, although tends to focus on own activity				
• Does not show awareness of others in the group unless close one-to-one attention is experienced				
6. Communication skills	P	E	S	R
• Is aware of appropriate interaction, can chat coherently and is able to use complex language skills				
• Body language may be inappropriate and may not always be coherent, but can use simple language skills		✓		
• Responses to verbal interaction may be mainly through body language; comprehension is limited				
• Can only respond to direct physical contact from others through touch, eye contact or facial expression				
7. Practical activities (craft, domestic chores, gardening)	P	E	S	R
• Can plan to carry out an activity, hold the goal in mind and work through a familiar sequence; may need help solving problems				
• More interested in the making or doing than the end result, needs prompting to remember purpose, can get distracted		✓		
• Activities need to be broken down and presented one step at a time, multisensory stimulation can help hold the attention				
• Unable to 'do' activities, but responds to the close contact of others and experiencing physical sensations				
8. Use of objects	P	E	S	R
• Plans to use and looks for objects that are not visible; may struggle if objects are not in usual/familiar places (e.g. toiletries in a bathroom cupboard)				
• Selects objects appropriately only if in view (e.g. toiletries on a shelf next to the washbasin)		✓		
• Randomly uses objects as chances on them; may use appropriately				
• May grip objects when placed in the hand but will not attempt to use them				

9. Looking at a newspaper/magazine	P	E	S	R
• Comprehends and shows interest in the content, turns the pages and looks at headlines and pictures				
• Turns the pages randomly, only attending to items pointed out by others		✓		
• Will hold and may feel the paper, but will not turn the pages unless directed and will not show interest in the content				
• May grip the paper if it is placed in the hand but may not be able to release the grip; or may not take hold of the paper				
NB: If the totals are evenly divided between activity levels, assume that the person is at the lower level but has the potential to move into the higher level. **Totals**	0	9	0	0

The Activity Level identified for this person is: Exploratory

Transfer this information to the front of the form.

Now use the relevant PAL Activity Profile to assist you to plan how you will help the person with their activities.

CASE STUDY 3

George Owen is a 45-year-old man with learning disability and early onset Alzheimer's disease. He lives in a small-group-living home, but he is beginning to increasingly rely on the support workers for all of his personal care needs. George is only able to carry out activities if the support worker guides him through the steps involved. When George is getting dressed, he needs to be offered clothing items, one at a time, although he is then able to put on some items if someone talks him through the activity. When George has a bath, he relies on support workers to do everything, only wiping his face and hands with the cloth with their encouragement.

George used to be a very caring and outgoing person, but now, although he watches the other residents, he does not make the first move to interact with them. When George's friends seek him out, he responds readily, although his understanding of their conversation seems limited and his response is mainly with a big smile and head nodding rather than with words. George's greatest enjoyment seems to be his mealtimes, and when seated with his friends he will laugh when he hears them laughing. However, most of his attention is focused on his meal, which he eats, using his hands, with great relish.

George used to spend his evenings playing pool with his friends, but this has become difficult because he does not follow the rules of the game and will walk off with the cue. This causes arguments with his friends and George began to spend more time alone, pacing the rooms and picking up items belonging to other residents. When the support workers noticed this, they began to spend more time strolling with him and encouraging him to pick up items that are not contentious. The support workers have noticed that George likes to feel the objects he picks up and that he is drawn to ones with soft textures. They have begun to spend individual time with George, but although they offer to look at the newspaper with him, he seems more interested in the feel of the paper than the content. George does show that he enjoys sitting, holding hands while they listen together to his favourite music.

When the Pool Activity Level (PAL) Checklist is completed for George it reveals that he is able to carry out activities at a *sensory* activity level. It is now possible to use this information in the Activity Profile to help George to use his remaining abilities and to compensate for his disabilities.

QCS POOL ACTIVITY LEVEL (PAL) CHECKLIST

Name: George Owen

Date: 1 September 2022

Completed by: A care worker

> Activity Level indicated: Sensory

Ensure you are familiar with the instructions before completion

Completing the Checklist	Key
• Thinking of the last two weeks, tick the statement that represents the person's ability in each section.	P = Planned level of ability
• If in doubt about which statement to tick, choose the level of ability that represents their average performance over the last two weeks.	E = Exploratory level of ability S = Sensory level of ability
• There should only be ONE TICK for each section.	R = Reflex level of ability
• You must tick one statement for each section.	
• Total the ticks at the bottom of each column over page.	

1. Bathing/Washing	P	E	S	R
• Can bathe/wash independently, sometimes with a little help to start				
• Needs soap put on flannel and one-step-at-a-time directions to wash				
• Mainly relies on others but will wipe own face and hands if encouraged			✓	
• Totally dependent and needs full assistance to wash or bathe				

2. Getting dressed	P	E	S	R
• Plans what to wear, selects own clothing from the cupboards; dresses in correct order				
• Needs help to plan what to wear but recognizes items and how to wear them; needs help with order of dressing				
• Needs help to plan and with order of dressing, but can carry out small activities if someone directs each step			✓	
• Totally dependent on someone to plan, sequence and complete dressing; may move limbs to assist				

3. Eating	P	E	S	R
• Eats independently and using the correct cutlery				
• Eats using a spoon and/or needs food to be cut up into small pieces				
• Only uses fingers to eat food			✓	
• Relies on others to be fed				

4. Contact with others	P	E	S	R
• Initiates social contact and responds to the needs of others				
• Aware of others and will seek interaction, but may be more concerned with own needs				
• Aware of others but waits for others to make the first social contact			✓	
• May not show an awareness of the presence of others unless in direct physical contact				

5. Groupwork skills	P	E	S	R
• Engages with others in a group activity, can take turns with the activity/tools				
• Occasionally engages with others in a group, moving in and out of the group at a whim				
• Aware of others in the group and will work alongside others, although tends to focus on own activity			✓	
• Does not show awareness of others in the group unless close one-to-one attention is experienced				

6. Communication skills	P	E	S	R
• Is aware of appropriate interaction, can chat coherently and is able to use complex language skills				
• Body language may be inappropriate and may not always be coherent, but can use simple language skills				
• Responses to verbal interaction may be mainly through body language; comprehension is limited			✓	
• Can only respond to direct physical contact from others through touch, eye contact or facial expression				

7. Practical activities (craft, domestic chores, gardening)	P	E	S	R
• Can plan to carry out an activity, hold the goal in mind and work through a familiar sequence; may need help solving problems				
• More interested in the making or doing than the end result, needs prompting to remember purpose, can get distracted				
• Activities need to be broken down and presented one step at a time, multisensory stimulation can help hold the attention			✓	
• Unable to 'do' activities, but responds to the close contact of others and experiencing physical sensations				

8. Use of objects	P	E	S	R
• Plans to use and looks for objects that are not visible; may struggle if objects are not in usual/familiar places (e.g. toiletries in a bathroom cupboard)				
• Selects objects appropriately only if in view (e.g. toiletries on a shelf next to the washbasin)				
• Randomly uses objects as chances on them; may use appropriately			✓	
• May grip objects when placed in the hand but will not attempt to use them				

9. Looking at a newspaper/magazine	P	E	S	R
• Comprehends and shows interest in the content, turns the pages and looks at headlines and pictures				
• Turns the pages randomly, only attending to items pointed out by others				
• Will hold and may feel the paper, but will not turn the pages unless directed and will not show interest in the content			✓	
• May grip the paper if it is placed in the hand but may not be able to release the grip; or may not take hold of the paper				
NB: If the totals are evenly divided between activity levels, assume that the person is at the lower level but has the potential to move into the higher level. **Totals**	0	0	9	0

The Activity Level identified for this person is: Sensory

Transfer this information to the front of the form.

> Now use the relevant PAL Activity Profile to assist you to plan how you will help the person with their activities.

CASE STUDY 4

Gertie Lawson lives in a nursing home. She has severe dementia caused by a combination of Alzheimer's disease and vascular disease that has resulted in her experiencing a series of strokes. Gertie relies on the nursing staff for all her care needs. Gertie does not seem to understand anything that is said to her and most of her contact with others is with people who come up close to her, when she will screw up the muscles of her face and gaze into their eyes. The nursing staff enable her to sit in the group singing activities, and she does become more animated when the music is playing, although she does not seem to be aware of the other group members unless those nearest to her are holding her hands. Gertie will also grasp firmly anything that is placed into the palm of her hands and sometimes she has trouble letting go again.

Gertie loves to see children and animals and will make crooning noises when they visit the ward. She dislikes loud, sudden noises and will shout angrily if they disturb her. Gertie used to work in a flower shop and she loves to look at, and smell, flowers when they are brought to her.

The nursing staff want to help Gertie to engage with her surroundings as much as she can. When the Pool Activity Level (PAL) Checklist is completed for Gertie it reveals that she is able to carry out activities at a *reflex* activity level. It is now possible to use this information in the Activity Profile to help Gertie to use her remaining abilities and to compensate for her disabilities.

QCS POOL ACTIVITY LEVEL (PAL) CHECKLIST

Name: Gertie Lawson

Date: 1 September 2022

Completed by: A care worker

> ### Activity Level indicated: Reflex

Ensure you are familiar with the instructions before completion

Completing the Checklist	Key
• Thinking of the last two weeks, tick the statement that represents the person's ability in each section. • If in doubt about which statement to tick, choose the level of ability that represents their average performance over the last two weeks. • There should only be ONE TICK for each section. • You must tick one statement for each section. • Total the ticks at the bottom of each column over page.	P = Planned level of ability E = Exploratory level of ability S = Sensory level of ability R = Reflex level of ability

1. Bathing/Washing	P	E	S	R
• Can bathe/wash independently, sometimes with a little help to start				
• Needs soap put on flannel and one-step-at-a-time directions to wash				
• Mainly relies on others but will wipe own face and hands if encouraged				
• Totally dependent and needs full assistance to wash or bathe				✓

2. Getting dressed	P	E	S	R
• Plans what to wear, selects own clothing from the cupboards; dresses in correct order				
• Needs help to plan what to wear but recognizes items and how to wear them; needs help with order of dressing				
• Needs help to plan and with order of dressing, but can carry out small activities if someone directs each step				
• Totally dependent on someone to plan, sequence and complete dressing; may move limbs to assist				✓

3. Eating	P	E	S	R
• Eats independently and using the correct cutlery				
• Eats using a spoon and/or needs food to be cut up into small pieces				
• Only uses fingers to eat food				
• Relies on others to be fed				✓

4. Contact with others	P	E	S	R
• Initiates social contact and responds to the needs of others				
• Aware of others and will seek interaction, but may be more concerned with own needs				
• Aware of others but waits for others to make the first social contact				
• May not show an awareness of the presence of others unless in direct physical contact				✓
5. Groupwork skills	**P**	**E**	**S**	**R**
• Engages with others in a group activity, can take turns with the activity/tools				
• Occasionally engages with others in a group, moving in and out of the group at a whim				
• Aware of others in the group and will work alongside others, although tends to focus on own activity				
• Does not show awareness of others in the group unless close one-to-one attention is experienced				✓
6. Communication skills	**P**	**E**	**S**	**R**
• Is aware of appropriate interaction, can chat coherently and is able to use complex language skills				
• Body language may be inappropriate and may not always be coherent, but can use simple language skills				
• Responses to verbal interaction may be mainly through body language; comprehension is limited				
• Can only respond to direct physical contact from others through touch, eye contact or facial expression				✓
7. Practical activities (craft, domestic chores, gardening)	**P**	**E**	**S**	**R**
• Can plan to carry out an activity, hold the goal in mind and work through a familiar sequence; may need help solving problems				
• More interested in the making or doing than the end result, needs prompting to remember purpose, can get distracted				
• Activities need to be broken down and presented one step at a time, multisensory stimulation can help hold the attention				
• Unable to 'do' activities, but responds to the close contact of others and experiencing physical sensations				✓
8. Use of objects	**P**	**E**	**S**	**R**
• Plans to use and looks for objects that are not visible; may struggle if objects are not in usual/familiar places (e.g. toiletries in a bathroom cupboard)				
• Selects objects appropriately only if in view (e.g. toiletries on a shelf next to the washbasin)				
• Randomly uses objects as chances on them; may use appropriately				
• May grip objects when placed in the hand but will not attempt to use them				✓

✓

9. Looking at a newspaper/magazine	P	E	S	R
• Comprehends and shows interest in the content, turns the pages and looks at headlines and pictures				
• Turns the pages randomly, only attending to items pointed out by others				
• Will hold and may feel the paper, but will not turn the pages unless directed and will not show interest in the content				
• May grip the paper if it is placed in the hand but may not be able to release the grip; or may not take hold of the paper				✓
NB: If the totals are evenly divided between activity levels, assume that the person is at the lower level but has the potential to move into the higher level. **Totals**	0	0	0	9

The Activity Level identified for this person is: Reflex

Transfer this information to the front of the form.

> Now use the relevant PAL Activity Profile to assist you to plan how you will help the person with their activities.

CASE STUDY 5

Ken Atkins lives in a residential home for people with dementia. He has frontal-temporal dementia, which is affecting his social behaviour and his ability to plan and to carry out some activities.

Ken is a retired bus driver and enjoys the outings on the minibus from the home. He always sits at the front and says he enjoys 'helping the ladies'. He chats to each person as they get on and off the bus, although occasionally his conversation becomes muddled. Ken is sometimes over-familiar and the activities coordinator needs to step in when his behaviour becomes inappropriate.

Ken is independent when getting washed but he usually needs reminding to do so. He also needs guidance with selecting the right clothes for the occasion and may not understand, for example, the need to dress warmly in the winter.

Ken enjoys eating and is always the first person into the dining room. He is independent in dining and also interacts well with others at his table, assisting them if needed, and starting conversations. Sometimes though, Ken gets too close to others and invades their personal space. This can cause arguments and Ken cannot see why others have reacted negatively.

Ken enjoys his daily after-breakfast routine of reading the *Daily Mail* newspaper with a coffee. He likes to read out points of interest to the care home staff and also to read them their horoscopes.

There is a gardening group at the home and Ken always joins in. He has always been a keen vegetable gardener and is able to draw on his skills and experience to lead gardening projects. However, he can become frustrated when he cannot see the gardening tools that he needs, as he will only use ones that are on the bench in front of him.

When the Pool Activity Level (PAL) Checklist is completed for Ken it reveals that he is able to carry out most activities at a *planned* activity level. However, Ken's ability in getting dressed, communicating with others and when using objects is at an *exploratory* activity level. It is now possible to use this information in the Activity Profile to help Ken to use his remaining abilities and to compensate for his disabilities.

QCS POOL ACTIVITY LEVEL (PAL) CHECKLIST

Name: Ken Atkins

Date: 1 September 2022

Completed by: A care worker

> Activity Level indicated: Planned

Ensure you are familiar with the instructions before completion

Completing the Checklist	Key
• Thinking of the last two weeks, tick the statement that represents the person's ability in each section.	P = Planned level of ability
• If in doubt about which statement to tick, choose the level of ability that represents their average performance over the last two weeks.	E = Exploratory level of ability S = Sensory level of ability
• There should only be ONE TICK for each section.	R = Reflex level of ability
• You must tick one statement for each section.	
• Total the ticks at the bottom of each column over page.	

1. Bathing/Washing	P	E	S	R
• Can bathe/wash independently, sometimes with a little help to start	✓			
• Needs soap put on flannel and one-step-at-a-time directions to wash				
• Mainly relies on others but will wipe own face and hands if encouraged				
• Totally dependent and needs full assistance to wash or bathe				

2. Getting dressed	P	E	S	R
• Plans what to wear, selects own clothing from the cupboards; dresses in correct order				
• Needs help to plan what to wear but recognizes items and how to wear them; needs help with order of dressing		✓		
• Needs help to plan and with order of dressing, but can carry out small activities if someone directs each step				
• Totally dependent on someone to plan, sequence and complete dressing; may move limbs to assist				

3. Eating	P	E	S	R
• Eats independently and using the correct cutlery	✓			
• Eats using a spoon and/or needs food to be cut up into small pieces				
• Only uses fingers to eat food				
• Relies on others to be fed				

4. Contact with others	P	E	S	R
• Initiates social contact and responds to the needs of others	✓			
• Aware of others and will seek interaction, but may be more concerned with own needs				
• Aware of others but waits for others to make the first social contact				
• May not show an awareness of the presence of others unless in direct physical contact				

5. Groupwork skills	P	E	S	R
• Engages with others in a group activity, can take turns with the activity/tools	✓			
• Occasionally engages with others in a group, moving in and out of the group at a whim				
• Aware of others in the group and will work alongside others, although tends to focus on own activity				
• Does not show awareness of others in the group unless close one-to-one attention is experienced				

6. Communication skills	P	E	S	R
• Is aware of appropriate interaction, can chat coherently and is able to use complex language skills				
• Body language may be inappropriate and may not always be coherent, but can use simple language skills		✓		
• Responses to verbal interaction may be mainly through body language; comprehension is limited				
• Can only respond to direct physical contact from others through touch, eye contact or facial expression				

7. Practical activities (craft, domestic chores, gardening)	P	E	S	R
• Can plan to carry out an activity, hold the goal in mind and work through a familiar sequence; may need help solving problems	✓			
• More interested in the making or doing than the end result, needs prompting to remember purpose, can get distracted				
• Activities need to be broken down and presented one step at a time, multisensory stimulation can help hold the attention				
• Unable to 'do' activities, but responds to the close contact of others and experiencing physical sensations				

8. Use of objects	P	E	S	R
• Plans to use and looks for objects that are not visible; may struggle if objects are not in usual/familiar places (e.g. toiletries in a bathroom cupboard)				
• Selects objects appropriately only if in view (e.g. toiletries on a shelf next to the washbasin)		✓		
• Randomly uses objects as chances on them; may use appropriately				
• May grip objects when placed in the hand but will not attempt to use them				

✓

9. Looking at a newspaper/magazine	P	E	S	R
• Comprehends and shows interest in the content, turns the pages and looks at headlines and pictures	✓			
• Turns the pages randomly, only attending to items pointed out by others				
• Will hold and may feel the paper, but will not turn the pages unless directed and will not show interest in the content				
• May grip the paper if it is placed in the hand but may not be able to release the grip; or may not take hold of the paper				
NB: If the totals are evenly divided between activity levels, assume that the person is at the lower level but has the potential to move into the higher level. **Totals**	6	3	0	0

The Activity Level identified for this person is: Planned

Transfer this information to the front of the form.

> Now use the relevant PAL Activity Profile to assist you to plan how you will help the person with their activities.

CASE STUDY 6

Irene Johnson is a retired nurse who came to London from the West Indies in 1955. She developed Alzheimer's disease six years ago and was being looked after at home by her husband. He was finding it difficult because Irene was not sleeping and frequently left the house and got lost. Irene now lives in a nearby specialist dementia care home and her husband visits her every day.

Irene relies on help from the care staff to get washed and dressed but will carry out small actions, such as drying her hands and fastening buttons, when the care team prompt her.

Irene is constantly moving around the home and will not sit down for meals. However, she will eat sandwiches and soft fruit as she walks around. As she walks around, Irene will pick up objects and put them into her pockets. Sometimes she puts them down the toilet, so staff and her husband are usually on stand-by to intervene.

Irene likes to go into the office with the staff and will have a cup of tea with them when they are having a meeting. She smiles when they talk and laugh, but only occasionally will answer direct questions with 'yes' or 'no'. Irene comes and goes in these meetings.

She does not participate in any of the organized activities in the home, but will often go into the sensory room and touch the objects in there and make appreciative vocal noises. Irene is particularly attracted to the bubble tube and will gaze at it for long periods of time.

Irene's husband brings her treats from home and will often bring in photo albums and holiday brochures of the West Indies. She will turn the pages randomly if he hands these to her, but will look more closely if he does this with her and points out the content.

When the Pool Activity Level (PAL) Checklist is completed for Irene it reveals that she is able to carry out most activities at a *sensory* activity level. However, when she is engaging with others and when she is engaging in the familiar activity of looking at a newspaper, Irene has a higher *exploratory* activity level of ability. It is now possible to use this information in the Activity Profile to help Irene to use her remaining abilities and to compensate for her disabilities.

✓

QCS POOL ACTIVITY LEVEL (PAL) CHECKLIST

Name: Irene Johnson

Date: 1 September 2022

Completed by: A care worker

> Activity Level indicated: Sensory

Ensure you are familiar with the instructions before completion

Completing the Checklist	Key
• Thinking of the last two weeks, tick the statement that represents the person's ability in each section.	P = Planned level of ability
	E = Exploratory level of ability
• If in doubt about which statement to tick, choose the level of ability that represents their average performance over the last two weeks.	S = Sensory level of ability
	R = Reflex level of ability
• There should only be ONE TICK for each section.	
• You must tick one statement for each section.	
• Total the ticks at the bottom of each column over page.	

1. Bathing/Washing	P	E	S	R
• Can bathe/wash independently, sometimes with a little help to start				
• Needs soap put on flannel and one-step-at-a-time directions to wash				
• Mainly relies on others but will wipe own face and hands if encouraged			✓	
• Totally dependent and needs full assistance to wash or bathe				
2. Getting dressed	**P**	**E**	**S**	**R**
• Plans what to wear, selects own clothing from the cupboards; dresses in correct order				
• Needs help to plan what to wear but recognizes items and how to wear them; needs help with order of dressing				
• Needs help to plan and with order of dressing, but can carry out small activities if someone directs each step			✓	
• Totally dependent on someone to plan, sequence and complete dressing; may move limbs to assist				
3. Eating	**P**	**E**	**S**	**R**
• Eats independently and using the correct cutlery				
• Eats using a spoon and/or needs food to be cut up into small pieces				
• Only uses fingers to eat food			✓	
• Relies on others to be fed				

4. Contact with others	P	E	S	R
• Initiates social contact and responds to the needs of others				
• Aware of others and will seek interaction, but may be more concerned with own needs				
• Aware of others but waits for others to make the first social contact			✓	
• May not show an awareness of the presence of others unless in direct physical contact				

5. Groupwork skills	P	E	S	R
• Engages with others in a group activity, can take turns with the activity/tools				
• Occasionally engages with others in a group, moving in and out of the group at a whim		✓		
• Aware of others in the group and will work alongside others, although tends to focus on own activity				
• Does not show awareness of others in the group unless close one-to-one attention is experienced				

6. Communication skills	P	E	S	R
• Is aware of appropriate interaction, can chat coherently and is able to use complex language skills				
• Body language may be inappropriate and may not always be coherent, but can use simple language skills				
• Responses to verbal interaction may be mainly through body language; comprehension is limited			✓	
• Can only respond to direct physical contact from others through touch, eye contact or facial expression				

7. Practical activities (craft, domestic chores, gardening)	P	E	S	R
• Can plan to carry out an activity, hold the goal in mind and work through a familiar sequence; may need help solving problems				
• More interested in the making or doing than the end result, needs prompting to remember purpose, can get distracted				
• Activities need to be broken down and presented one step at a time, multisensory stimulation can help hold the attention			✓	
• Unable to 'do' activities, but responds to the close contact of others and experiencing physical sensations				

8. Use of objects	P	E	S	R
• Plans to use and looks for objects that are not visible; may struggle if objects are not in usual/familiar places (e.g. toiletries in a bathroom cupboard)				
• Selects objects appropriately only if in view (e.g. toiletries on a shelf next to the washbasin)				
• Randomly uses objects as chances on them; may use appropriately			✓	
• May grip objects when placed in the hand but will not attempt to use them				

✓

9. Looking at a newspaper/magazine	P	E	S	R
• Comprehends and shows interest in the content, turns the pages and looks at headlines and pictures				
• Turns the pages randomly, only attending to items pointed out by others		✓		
• Will hold and may feel the paper, but will not turn the pages unless directed and will not show interest in the content				
• May grip the paper if it is placed in the hand but may not be able to release the grip; or may not take hold of the paper				
NB: If the totals are evenly divided between activity levels, assume that the person is at the lower level but has the potential to move into the higher level. **Totals**	0	2	7	0

The Activity Level identified for this person is: Sensory

Transfer this information to the front of the form.

> Now use the relevant PAL Activity Profile to assist you to plan how you will help the person with their activities.

CASE STUDY 7

Millie Dunbar had been living at home with some support from her neighbours. She has no relatives and had refused help from her social services department. Millie was found on the floor by a neighbour and was admitted initially to the Accident and Emergency ward to treat her dehydration and minor injuries from her fall. She was then admitted to the dementia assessment ward of the community hospital.

Millie is able to carry out personal care activities if the nurses guide her by breaking down each activity into single steps. She can wash and dress herself when these activities are broken down in this way and if the objects she needs are in her view. Otherwise Millie becomes muddled and moves on to do something else.

Millie can manage to eat her meals using a spoon and fork. Staff need to cut her food up so that she can manage this. At the dining table, Millie glances at others when they make noises or touch her, but she does not initiate any interaction and tends to focus on her meal, leaving the table as soon as she has finished. When others try to engage Millie in conversation, she will chat but her use of spoken language is limited, although she uses a large amount of tone and facial expression to show how she is feeling.

Millie is attending occupational therapy sessions as part of her assessment to determine her needs and ability to live at home. The occupational therapist (OT) has included Millie in some group activities, but has found that Millie does not respond to group aims and prefers to only focus on the activity. In a one-to-one newspaper activity, where the aim is to increase a patient's orientation to current events and time, the OT has observed that Millie enjoys crumpling the newspaper rather than following the content.

When the Pool Activity Level (PAL) Checklist is completed for Millie it reveals that she is able to carry out most activities at an *exploratory* activity level. However, there is almost an even split between this level and the *sensory* activity level. As the number of ticks is almost evenly divided between these two activity levels, the staff assume that Millie is currently functioning at the lower level of ability for the purpose of selecting the Activity Profile, but they are aware that they need to offer her the opportunity to move into the higher level of ability.

Staff also create an Individual Action Plan for Millie to assist her with the activities of dressing, bathing and dining. Millie's ability in each of these activities has been revealed on the PAL Checklist as at an *exploratory* activity level and this plan will ensure that, for these activities, Millie is given the opportunity to maintain her current skills at the higher level than for her general profile.

QCS POOL ACTIVITY LEVEL (PAL) CHECKLIST

Name: Millie Dunbar

Date: 1 September 2022

Completed by: A care worker

> Activity Level indicated: Sensory

Ensure you are familiar with the instructions before completion

Completing the Checklist	Key
• Thinking of the last two weeks, tick the statement that represents the person's ability in each section.	P = Planned level of ability
	E = Exploratory level of ability
• If in doubt about which statement to tick, choose the level of ability that represents their average performance over the last two weeks.	S = Sensory level of ability
	R = Reflex level of ability
• There should only be ONE TICK for each section.	
• You must tick one statement for each section.	
• Total the ticks at the bottom of each column over page.	

1. Bathing/Washing	P	E	S	R
• Can bathe/wash independently, sometimes with a little help to start				
• Needs soap put on flannel and one-step-at-a-time directions to wash		✓		
• Mainly relies on others but will wipe own face and hands if encouraged				
• Totally dependent and needs full assistance to wash or bathe				
2. Getting dressed	**P**	**E**	**S**	**R**
• Plans what to wear, selects own clothing from the cupboards; dresses in correct order				
• Needs help to plan what to wear but recognizes items and how to wear them; needs help with order of dressing		✓		
• Needs help to plan and with order of dressing, but can carry out small activities if someone directs each step				
• Totally dependent on someone to plan, sequence and complete dressing; may move limbs to assist				
3. Eating	**P**	**E**	**S**	**R**
• Eats independently and using the correct cutlery				
• Eats using a spoon and/or needs food to be cut up into small pieces		✓		
• Only uses fingers to eat food				
• Relies on others to be fed				

4. Contact with others	P	E	S	R
• Initiates social contact and responds to the needs of others				
• Aware of others and will seek interaction, but may be more concerned with own needs				
• Aware of others but waits for others to make the first social contact			✓	
• May not show an awareness of the presence of others unless in direct physical contact				

5. Groupwork skills	P	E	S	R
• Engages with others in a group activity, can take turns with the activity/tools				
• Occasionally engages with others in a group, moving in and out of the group at a whim				
• Aware of others in the group and will work alongside others, although tends to focus on own activity			✓	
• Does not show awareness of others in the group unless close one-to-one attention is experienced				

6. Communication skills	P	E	S	R
• Is aware of appropriate interaction, can chat coherently and is able to use complex language skills				
• Body language may be inappropriate and may not always be coherent, but can use simple language skills		✓		
• Responses to verbal interaction may be mainly through body language; comprehension is limited				
• Can only respond to direct physical contact from others through touch, eye contact or facial expression				

7. Practical activities (craft, domestic chores, gardening)	P	E	S	R
• Can plan to carry out an activity, hold the goal in mind and work through a familiar sequence; may need help solving problems				
• More interested in the making or doing than the end result, needs prompting to remember purpose, can get distracted				
• Activities need to be broken down and presented one step at a time, multisensory stimulation can help hold the attention			✓	
• Unable to 'do' activities, but responds to the close contact of others and experiencing physical sensations				

8. Use of objects	P	E	S	R
• Plans to use and looks for objects that are not visible; may struggle if objects are not in usual/familiar places (e.g. toiletries in a bathroom cupboard)				
• Selects objects appropriately only if in view (e.g. toiletries on a shelf next to the washbasin)		✓		
• Randomly uses objects as chances on them; may use appropriately				
• May grip objects when placed in the hand but will not attempt to use them				

9. Looking at a newspaper/magazine	P	E	S	R
• Comprehends and shows interest in the content, turns the pages and looks at headlines and pictures				
• Turns the pages randomly, only attending to items pointed out by others				
• Will hold and may feel the paper, but will not turn the pages unless directed and will not show interest in the content			✓	
• May grip the paper if it is placed in the hand but may not be able to release the grip; or may not take hold of the paper				
NB: If the totals are evenly divided between activity levels, assume that the person is at the lower level but has the potential to move into the higher level. **Totals**	0	5	4	0

The Activity Level identified for this person is: Sensory

Transfer this information to the front of the form.

> Now use the relevant PAL Activity Profile to assist you to plan how you will help the person with their activities.

These case studies give examples of how the behaviour of the person can be recorded to identify the level of ability using the PAL Checklist. The user of the PAL Instrument is then prompted to select the appropriate PAL Activity Profile to act as a general guide to engaging with the person in a variety of activities. Including the information gained from the person's Life History Profile enhances this information.

In addition to the general PAL Activity Profile, the user is also able to complete a PAL Individual Action Plan, which acts as a specific guide to facilitating personal activities.

In the first four case studies, the level of ability in each task on the Checklist is the same throughout. Therefore completion of the Individual Action Plan would use the same level of ability information for all three personal care tasks. In the final three case studies, the person is functioning at different levels of ability in different activities. The Individual Action Plan would reflect this by having a record of how to engage the person in the activities at the relevant level of ability as revealed by the checklist. An example of how to complete the Individual Action Plan in these circumstances is given in Chapter 8.

PLANNING INTERVENTIONS

Completing the PAL Activity Profile and the PAL Individual Action Plan

When a caregiver helps a person with cognitive impairment to carry out an activity it is important that they do not do too much because this will undermine the person's self-confidence and could result in the person becoming more dependent. Equally, it is important that caregivers do not do too little because the well-being of the person will be undermined as they struggle to meet the demands of the activity. It is therefore helpful to plan the best way of facilitating the person with cognitive impairments to carry out activities. Staff in residential homes will be familiar with care plans, although these sometimes focus on the tasks to be done rather than on the method of helping the person to carry them out. Although planning caregiving in a person's own home where a family member, for example, is the carer might seem excessive, it is essential in clarifying the most effective way of enabling the person being cared for. Planning in this way also promotes a consistent approach from all caregivers, whether they are staff, relatives or friends.

THE PAL ACTIVITY PROFILE

This Profile assists caregivers in translating an understanding of the level of ability of the person with cognitive impairment into practical methods of helping them to engage in activities. There are four Activity Profiles, one for each activity level. The caregiver should select the Profile which is revealed as appropriate following completion of the PAL Checklist. Each Profile describes how to assist the person by positioning objects that are needed to carry out the activity and by giving verbal or physical directions. The objectives and characteristics of activities that are likely to be meaningful to a person at the level of ability are also described in each Profile.

In addition, some information about the person's likely abilities and limitations are given. This can be helpful in aiding the caregiver to build on the person's strengths and to compensate for their limitations.

The following pages demonstrate how the PAL Activity Profile can be used to help the person to undertake a range of activities and thus to maintain a stimulating and fulfilling life.

The Profile describes how, in general, to help a person with cognitive impairment at different levels of ability. The final stage of using the PAL Activity Profile is to work out what activities should be provided or encouraged. This information is entered in the final box on the Profile form. Chapter 6 describes how to use the information from the Life History Profile to ensure that activities that are meaningful to the person are entered on this form.

In the Checklist examples (see Chapter 7), John is at a *planned* activity level of ability. As the PAL Activity Profile reveals, this means that he can explore different ways of carrying out an activity and can carry out activities as long as the objects he needs are in their usual place and the end result of the activity is obvious, so he knows what he is working towards and when he has finished. However, John may not be able to solve any problems that arise and, for example, may not be able to look for any objects that he needs to carry out the activity if they are not where he expects to find them.

The Profile for Elsie reveals that she can carry out very familiar activities in very familiar environments, but may have a problem with those that involve a complex series of stages, such as getting dressed. So although she is completing the activity of getting dressed, and wishes to do this alone, she is not able to carry out the steps involved in the correct sequence and therefore the end result is haphazard. Elsie also tends to start activities but not finish them and this may be because she has difficulty fixing an end result in her mind at the beginning.

The Checklist example for George reveals that he is able to carry out activities at a *sensory* activity level of ability. The Profile indicates that, at this level of ability, George is likely to be responding to bodily sensations rather than engaging in the 'doing' of activities. Any activities he is helped to carry out successfully will be those that are simple one-step ones, or those that have been broken down into single stages. At this level, George is likely to be limited in his ability to initiate social contact and will be reliant on others making the first move.

Gertie only engages with her surroundings when there is a direct impact on her own senses; she does not actively seek engagement and so is very reliant on others to ensure that she receives opportunities for stimulation and fulfilment. The Profile for Gertie's *reflex* activity level of ability shows that she can respond in a reflex way to direct sensory stimulation and through this she can become more aware of herself and her surroundings. At this level, Gertie may have difficulty attending to, or may become agitated by, complex and multiple sensory messages. Completion of the appropriate PAL Activity Profile will guide caregivers in presenting all activities that the person may wish to undertake in a way that maximizes the opportunity for meaningful engagement. The example Checklists are developed here so that the Profiles may be clarified.

THE PAL INDIVIDUAL ACTION PLAN

Caregivers often seek specific guidance for enabling the person they care for to realize their potential for carrying out personal care activities, such as bathing, dining or dressing. The PAL Individual Action Plan has been designed so that a person with cognitive impairment is facilitated to carry out a range of personal care activities using their abilities.

A person with cognitive impairment will have some cognitive skills that are still intact. This will vary depending on the area of damage in the brain. The ability to carry out activities, in any case, does not always rely on the integrity of the brain; familiarity with the activity and the activity environment, and the type of support the person receives while carrying out the activity, will either facilitate or undermine the person's ability. It is often apparent that a person does have different levels of ability in different activities. Completion of the PAL Checklist will reveal this.

In this manual version of the PAL Instrument, the caregiver is guided to note the level of ability of the person in the personal care activities of dressing, bathing and dining and to then refer to the Individual Action Plan guidance notes. These reveal a method for facilitating the person's engagement in each of the three activities.

Transferring the information from the guidance notes onto the Individual Action Plan can be done in several ways. The user can photocopy the guidance notes and then cut and stick them onto the Individual Action Plan, or the user may prefer to handwrite the information.

Because social and psychological factors also play an important role in determining an individual's ability to carry out an activity, the user is also encouraged to consider these when completing the Individual Action Plan. By referring to the person's Life History Profile and by observing the person's responses when assisting them to carry out an activity, it is possible to also pay attention to the person's preferences and to plan to accommodate these.

The digital version of the PAL Instrument (accessed for free at www.qcs.co.uk/digital-pool-activity-level-pal-instrument) automatically calculates the abilities of the individual and creates a comprehensive PAL Guide accordingly. The PAL Guide provides details of how to support the person at any of the four PAL levels of ability, across five everyday activities: dining, washing, dressing, interacting and engaging in leisure activities.

Blank copies of the PAL Instrument, including the Checklist, PAL Activity Profile, Individual Action Plan and Engagement Measure, can be found in Chapter 1 at the front of this book. They may be photocopied for your use with the people for whom you care.

QCS PAL ACTIVITY PROFILE

PLANNED ACTIVITY LEVEL OF ABILITY
Name: John Porter

Date: 1 September 2022

Likely abilities

- Can explore different ways of carrying out an activity
- Can work towards completing a task with a tangible result
- Can look in obvious places for any objects

Likely limitations

- May not be able to solve problems that arise
- May not be able to understand complex sentences
- May not search beyond the usual places for objects

Caregiver's role

- To enable the person to take control of the activity and master the steps involved
- To encourage the person to initiate social interactions
- To solve problems as they arise

Using the PAL Activity Profile to support the person

Position of objects	Ensure that objects and materials are in their usual, familiar places.
Verbal directions	Explain activity using short sentences by avoiding using connecting phrases such as 'and', 'but', 'therefore' or 'if'. Allow time for a response. Repeat the directions if the person is struggling to recall the guidance. Encourage the person to solve problems encountered through gentle prompts.
Demonstrated directions	Show the person how to avoid possible errors. If problems cannot be solved independently then demonstrate the solution. Encourage the person then to copy.
Working with others	The person is able to make the first contact and should be encouraged and be given opportunity to initiate social contact.
Activity characteristics	There is a goal or end product, with a set process, or 'recipe', to achieve it.

Suitable leisure activities

- Identify an activity of interest to the person based on knowledge of their interests, career, home life and so on, or select one of the activities suggested below as a starting point.
- Ensure the task you select is not overly complex.
- An element of competition with others is motivating.

– Memory games, newspapers, exercise activities, art/craft, board games, computer games, conversation, cooking, gardening, DIY, word quizzes/crosswords.

Activity plan:

Gardening

Stamp collecting

Social outings/dining out

Using the PAL Activity Profile to support John will help him to remain independent for as long as possible, given the nature of his condition, if his surroundings remain constant so that the familiar positioning of items will act as cues for the next stage in an activity. John will also be able to carry out less familiar activities so long as he is made aware of the aim of an activity and the methods made clear. This clarity will help John to feel confident and secure when he is carrying out activities so that his self-esteem will not be undermined.

The PAL Individual Action Plan can also be completed to guide caregivers in how best to support John's specific and unique personal care needs.

QCS PAL INDIVIDUAL ACTION PLAN

Name: John Porter

Date: 1 September 2022

DRESSING
Favourite garments
Tweed jacket

Preferred routine
Always wears a shirt, tie and jacket

Grooming likes and dislikes
Visits the barber every four weeks

Method

- Encourage John to plan what to wear and to select own clothes from the wardrobe.
- Encourage John to put on his own clothes; be available to assist if required.
- Point out labels on clothing to help orientate the back from the front.
- Encourage John to attend to grooming such as brushing hair and cleaning shoes.

BATHING/SHOWERING
Favourite toiletries
Gillette Sport range

Preferred routine
Has a shower every morning before breakfast. Has an evening bath two to three times a week

Bathing likes and dislikes
Likes having his back washed by his wife

Method

- Encourage John to plan when he will have the bath, to draw the water and to select toiletries from the usual cupboard or shelf.
- Encourage John to wash his own body; be available to assist if required.
- Encourage John to release the water afterwards and to wipe the bath.

DINING
Favourite foods
Indian, Italian and fine dining, malt whisky

✓

Preferred routine
Has muesli for breakfast while listening to the news on Radio 4. Has a light lunch and evening dinner. Has a whisky each evening before going to bed

Dining likes and dislikes
Expects high standards of restaurant service

Method

- Encourage John to select when and what he wishes to eat.
- Encourage John to prepare the dining table and to select the cutlery, crockery and condiments from the usual cupboards or drawers.
- Encourage John to clear away afterwards.

QCS PAL ACTIVITY PROFILE

EXPLORATORY ACTIVITY LEVEL OF ABILITY

Name: Elsie Jones

Date: 1 September 2022

Likely abilities

- Can carry out very familiar tasks in familiar surroundings
- Enjoys the experience of doing a task more than the end result
- Can carry out more complex tasks if they are broken down into two- to three-step stages

Likely limitations

- May not have an end result in mind when starts a task
- May not recognize when the task is completed
- Relies on cues such as diaries, newspaper, lists and labels

Caregiver's role

- To enable the person to experience the sensation of doing the activity rather than focusing on the end result
- To break the activity into manageable chunks
- To keep directions simple and understandable
- To approach and make first contact as it is rarely initiated by the person

Using the PAL Activity Profile to support the person

Position of objects	Ensure that objects and materials are in the line of vision.
Verbal directions	Explain task using short simple sentences. Avoid using connecting phrases such as 'and', 'but' or 'therefore'. Also avoid using prepositions such as 'in', 'by' or 'for'. Repeat the directions if the person is struggling to recall the guidance.
Demonstrated directions	Break the activity into two or three steps at a time.
Working with others	Others must approach the person and make the first contact.
Activity characteristics	There is no pressure to perform to a set of rules, or to achieve an end result. There is an element of creativity and spontaneity.

✓

Suitable leisure activities

- Identify an activity of interest to the person based on knowledge of their interests, career, home life and so on, or select one of the activities suggested below as a starting point.
  - Outings, newspaper discussions, exercise activities, art/craft, food tasting, board games, computer games, reminiscence objects, conversation, cooking, gardening, DIY, flower arranging.

Activity plan:

Arts and crafts

Fashion – shopping, looking at magazines, TV shows

Reminiscence

Beauty sessions – nails, make-up, hair

Using the PAL Activity Profile to support Elsie, the caregiver needs to guide Elsie to carry out any activities in stages. Elsie wishes to retain her independence in getting dressed, and at the same time return to her previous standard of grooming. The caregiver can facilitate this by helping her sort out her wardrobe and drawers so that items are kept together and are labelled. This may help Elsie to select garments appropriately. In addition, Elsie may enjoy the caregiver assisting her while she dresses, if the focus is on choosing what to wear and looking at the colours, patterns and texture of the clothes. This is likely to have more meaning to Elsie than the actual act of dressing. It will be important that the caregiver helps Elsie to make the finishing touches of hair combing, make-up and jewellery. Elsie can be reassured about her appearance by being encouraged to check herself in a mirror.

This information will help Elsie's family to enable Elsie to experience feelings of self-confidence and self-esteem, because she will be aware that her appearance meets her own standards, while at the same time her independence has not been taken away: she has been enabled to carry out the dressing task at her own level of ability.

The PAL Individual Action Plan can also be completed to guide caregivers in how best to support Elsie's specific and unique personal care needs.

QCS PAL INDIVIDUAL ACTION PLAN

Name: Elsie Jones

Date: 1 September 2022

DRESSING
Favourite garments
Pink Chanel blouse, Dior best dress

Preferred routine
Dresses after breakfast in casual clothes. Changes into smart clothes for evening meal

Grooming likes and dislikes
Wears full make-up every day and has to put it on before she meets anyone

Method

- Encourage discussion about the clothing to be worn for the day: is it suitable for the weather or the occasion? Is it a favourite item?
- Spend time colour-matching items of clothing and select accessories.
- Break down the activity into manageable chunks: help lay the clothes out in order so that underclothing is at the top of the pile. If she wishes to be helped, talk Elsie through the task: 'Put on your underclothes', 'Now put on your trousers/dress and blouse/cardigan.'
- Encourage Elsie to check her appearance in the mirror.

BATHING/SHOWERING
Favourite toiletries
Crabtree and Evelyn Rose soap, Chanel No. 5 perfume

Preferred routine
Has a bath every night before going to bed, and a wash in the morning

Bathing likes and dislikes
Likes a full bath with scented bath cream, enjoys a soak for about 15 minutes. Wants to be helped into the bath, then left on her own to bathe

Method

- Break down the activity into manageable chunks: suggest that Elsie fills the bath. When that is accomplished, suggest that she gathers together items such as soap, shampoo, flannel and towels.

- When Elsie is in the bath, suggest that she soaps and rinses her upper body. When that is accomplished, suggest that she soaps and rinses her lower body.
- Ensure that bathing items are on view and that containers are clearly labelled.
- Have attractive objects around the bathroom such as unusual bath oil bottles or shells and encourage discussion and exploration of them.

DINING

Favourite foods

Soup and sandwiches, sherry

Preferred routine

Enjoys breakfast in bed, main meal at lunch, hot chocolate in bed each night

Dining likes and dislikes

Likes to use a spoon to eat meals. Dislikes having a mug for drinks; prefers a china cup with a saucer

Method

- Store cutlery and crockery in view and encourage Elsie to select own tools for dining.
- Offer food using simple choices.
- Create a social atmosphere using table decorations and music, and promote conversation.

QCS PAL ACTIVITY PROFILE

SENSORY ACTIVITY LEVEL OF ABILITY
Name: George Owen
Date: 1 September 2022

Likely abilities

- Is likely to be responding to bodily sensations. Can be guided to carry out single-step activities
- Can carry out more complex activities if they are broken down into one step at a time

Likely limitations

- May not have any conscious plan to carry out a movement to achieve a particular end result
- May be relying on others to make social contact

Caregiver's role

- To enable the person to experience the effect of the activity on their senses
- To break the activity into one step at a time
- To keep directions simple and understandable
- To approach and make the first contact with the person

Using the PAL Activity Profile to support the person

Position of objects	Ensure that the person becomes aware of objects and materials by making bodily contact.
Verbal directions	Limit requests to carry out actions to the naming of the action and of the object involved, e.g. 'lift your arm', 'hold the brush'.
Demonstrated directions	Demonstrate to the person the action on the object. Break the activity down into one step at a time.
Working with others	Others must approach the person and make the first contact. Use touch and the person's name to sustain the social contact.
Activity characteristics	The activity is used as an opportunity for a sensory experience. This may be multisensory. Repetitive actions are appropriate.

Suitable leisure activities

- Identify an activity of interest to the person based on knowledge of their interests, career, home life and so on, or select one of the activities suggested below as a starting point.
  - Sensory box, smells, food tasting, hand massage, exercises, music and singing, dancing, sweeping, polishing, wiping tables and so on.

Activity plan:

Music – listening, playing instruments (tambourine, bells, maracas)

Sensory activities – sensory room, sensory box

Dining room attendant – wiping tables, sweeping floor

As we see in George's case study (see Chapter 7), George is engaging with his surroundings by enjoying the sensations, particularly of touch. The caregivers have recognized the importance of this to George and are providing him with opportunities for interacting with them through the medium of touch.

This PAL Activity Profile will help caregivers to also realize that it is important for George to enjoy being involved in the process of carrying out the activity, rather than in the end result. It will also help them to recognize that, despite his disability, George still has many abilities and that he can do activities which do not have more than one step. There are many such activities, including sweeping, polishing and wiping surfaces.

When activities are presented to George in this way, he is likely to regain his sense of being a part of things in his home and, by his actions, of being able to make things happen.

The PAL Individual Action Plan can also be completed to guide caregivers in how best to support George's specific and unique personal care needs.

QCS PAL INDIVIDUAL ACTION PLAN

Name: George Owen

Date: 1 September 2022

DRESSING
Favourite garments
Tracksuit and Manchester United T-shirts

Preferred routine
Get dressed before breakfast. Has Radio 1 playing

Grooming likes and dislikes
Doesn't like shaving and prefers to have a beard

Method

- Offer a simple choice of clothing to be worn.
- Spend a few moments enjoying the sensations of the clothing: feeling the fabric, gently rubbing George's hand over different textures, or smelling the clean laundry.
- Break down the task into one step at a time: 'Put on your vest', 'Now put on your pants', 'Now put on your trousers.'

BATHING/SHOWERING
Favourite toiletries
Manchester United liquid soap

Preferred routine
Washes every morning and has a bath once a week

Bathing likes and dislikes
Hates soap in his eyes

Method

- Prepare the bathroom and run the bath water for George.
- Make the bathroom warm and inviting – play music (Radio 1), use Manchester United bubble bath, have candles lit on a safely-out-of-reach shelf, have floating bath games.
- Break down the task into one step at a time and give George simple directions: 'Rub the soap on the cloth', 'Rub your arm', 'Rinse your arm', 'Rub your chest', 'Rinse your chest.'

DINING

Favourite foods
Sausage and mash, beef pie and chips

Preferred routine
Sits on his chair with the Manchester United cushion. Always eats with his friends. Uses his hands and uses wet wipes to clean them

Dining likes and dislikes
Doesn't like spicy food. Doesn't like being given a fork but will occasionally accept a spoon to eat with

Method

- Serve food so that it presents a variety of colours, tastes and textures.
- Offer George finger foods, encourage him to feel the food.
- Offer George a spoon, place it in his hand and direct him to 'Scoop the potato', 'Lift your arm', 'Open your mouth.'

QCS PAL ACTIVITY PROFILE

REFLEX ACTIVITY LEVEL OF ABILITY
Name: Gertie Lawson

Date: 1 September 2022

Likely abilities

- Can make reflex responses to direct sensory stimulation
- Direct sensory stimulation can increase awareness of self and others
- May respond to social engagement through the use of body language

Likely limitations

- May not be aware of the surrounding environment or even of their own body
- May have difficulty organizing the multiple sensations that are being experienced
- May become agitated in an environment that is over-stimulating

Caregiver's role

- To enable the person to be more aware of themselves
- To arouse the person to be more aware of their surroundings
- To engage with the person through direct sensory stimulation
- To monitor the environment and reduce multiple stimuli, loud noises and background sounds

Using the PAL Activity Profile to support the person

Position of objects	Direct stimuli to the area of body being targeted, e.g. stroke the person's arm before placing it in a sleeve. Use light across the person's field of vision to encourage eye movement.
Verbal directions	Limit spoken directions to movement directions, e.g. 'lift', 'hold', 'open'. Use a warm, reassuring tone and adapt volume to establish a connection with the person.
Demonstrated directions	Guide movements by touching the relevant body part.
Working with others	Maintain eye contact, make maximum use of facial expression, gestures and body posture for a non-verbal conversation. Use social actions which can be imitated, e.g. smiling, waving, shaking hands.
Activity characteristics	The activity focuses on a single sensation: touch, smell, sound, sight, taste.

Suitable leisure activities

- Identify an activity of interest to the person based on knowledge of their interests, career, home life and so on, or select one of the activities suggested below as a starting point.

✓

– Smells, food tasting, hand massage, music, lights, textured objects, chimes, sensory mobiles.

Activity plan:

Music appreciation – listening to favourite pieces, including listening to the visiting children's music group

Hand massage

Sensory activities

- handling strong colour and smelling flowers and herbs

- rainmaker

- sensory apron

Gertie's PAL Activity Profile reveals how important it is that others approach her and make contact with her by stimulating her sense of hearing, sight, smell, taste or touch. When this happens, Gertie obviously responds, so planning to make it happen frequently will give Gertie an increased opportunity for engaging with others and her surroundings.

The PAL Individual Action Plan can also be completed to guide caregivers in how best to support Gertie's specific and unique personal care needs.

QCS PAL INDIVIDUAL ACTION PLAN

Name: *Gertie Lawson*

Date: *1 September 2022*

DRESSING
Favourite garments
Soft wool cardigans and a knitted-squares blanket for her knees

Preferred routine
Gentle music and talking to her soothingly while helping her

Grooming likes and dislikes
Loves having her hair brushed

Method

- Prepare the clothing for Gertie, ensure the dressing area is private and that a chair or bed at the right height is available for sitting.
- Talk through each stage of the activity as you put the clothing onto Gertie, use a calm tone, speak slowly and smile to indicate that you are non-threatening.
- Stimulate a response in the limb being dressed by using firm but gentle stroking. Ask Gertie to assist you when necessary by using one-word requests: 'Lift', 'Stand', 'Sit.'
- At the end of dressing, spend some time brushing Gertie's hair using firm massaging brush strokes.

BATHING/SHOWERING
Favourite toiletries
Lavender bubble bath

Preferred routine
Sleeps well after a bath before going to bed

Bathing likes and dislikes
Dislikes having her hair washed in the bath but will accept it being done at the washbasin

Method

- Prepare the bathroom and run the bath water, put in lavender bubble bath.
- Ensure that the bathroom is warm and inviting and feels secure by closing the door and curtains and providing a slip-resistant bath mat in the bath and on the floor. Clear away any unnecessary items which may be confusing.
- Use firm, massaging movements when soaping and rinsing Gertie.

- Wrap her securely in a towel when she is out of the bath.

DINING

Favourite foods
Cake, soft fruits and chocolate

Preferred routine
Enjoys eating from a spoon with help

Dining likes and dislikes
Doesn't like to sit at the table with others, prefers to be helped to eat in her armchair

Method

- Use touch on Gertie's forearm to make contact, maintain eye contact, and smile to indicate the pleasure of the activity.
- Place a spoon in Gertie's hand. Close your hand over hers and raise the spoon with food on it to her mouth.
- As the food reaches Gertie's mouth say 'open' and open your own mouth to demonstrate. Touch Gertie's lips gently with the spoon.

QCS PAL ACTIVITY PROFILE

PLANNED ACTIVITY LEVEL OF ABILITY

Name: Ken Atkins

Date: 1 September 2022

Likely abilities

- Can explore different ways of carrying out an activity
- Can work towards completing a task with a tangible result
- Can look in obvious places for any objects

Likely limitations

- May not be able to solve problems that arise
- May not be able to understand complex sentences
- May not search beyond the usual places for objects

Caregiver's role

- To enable the person to take control of the activity and master the steps involved
- To encourage the person to initiate social interactions
- To solve problems as they arise

Using the PAL Activity Profile to support the person

Position of objects	Ensure that objects and materials are in their usual, familiar places.
Verbal directions	Explain activity using short sentences by avoiding using connecting phrases such as 'and', 'but', 'therefore' or 'if'. Allow time for a response. Repeat the directions if the person is struggling to recall the guidance. Encourage the person to solve problems encountered through gentle prompts.
Demonstrated directions	Show the person how to avoid possible errors. If problems cannot be solved independently then demonstrate the solution. Encourage the person then to copy.
Working with others	The person is able to make the first contact and should be encouraged and be given opportunity to initiate social contact.
Activity characteristics	There is a goal or end product, with a set process, or 'recipe', to achieve it.

Suitable leisure activities

- Identify an activity of interest to the person based on knowledge of their interests, career, home life and so on, or select one of the activities suggested below as a starting point.
- Ensure the task you select is not overly complex.

- An element of competition with others is motivating.
    - Memory games, newspapers, exercise activities, art/craft, board games, computer games, conversation, cooking, gardening, DIY, word quizzes/crosswords.

Activity plan:

Gardening

Social outings/dining

News group

Quizzes

Completion of the PAL Individual Action Plan will guide caregivers to enable Ken's level of ability by supporting his motivation to stay as independent as possible through a good understanding of his lifestyle preferences.

QCS PAL INDIVIDUAL ACTION PLAN

Name: Ken Atkins

Date: 1 September 2022

DRESSING
Favourite garments
Open collar shirt and trousers; jacket and tie for outings; cap for all outside events

Preferred routine
Has a cup of tea (milk, one sugar) in bed before getting up. Showers and dresses before breakfast

Grooming likes and dislikes
Always uses an electric shaver, dislikes wet shaving

Method

- Encourage discussion about the clothing to be worn for the day: is it suitable for the weather or the occasion, is it a favourite item?
- Spend time colour-matching items of clothing and select accessories.
- Break down the activity into manageable chunks: help lay the clothes out in order so that underclothing is at the top of the pile. If Ken wishes to be helped, talk him through the task: 'Put on your underclothes', 'Now put on your trousers and shirt.'
- Encourage Ken to check his appearance in the mirror.

BATHING/SHOWERING
Favourite toiletries
Lynx Africa shower gel and deodorant. Old Spice aftershave

Preferred routine
Shower in the morning, wash at night

Bathing likes and dislikes
Does not like having a bath

Method

- Encourage Ken to plan when he will have the shower, to turn on the shower and to select toiletries from the usual cupboard or shelf.
- Encourage Ken to wash his own body; be available to assist if required.
- Encourage Ken to turn off the shower, and to wipe the shower unit.

✓

DINING
Favourite foods
Fish and chips, roast dinners

Preferred routine
Likes to be the first into the dining room. Sits at the window table, facing the room. Prefers his main meal at lunch time and a light tea

Dining likes and dislikes
Doesn't like spicy food

Method

- Encourage Ken to select when and what he wishes to eat.
- Encourage Ken to prepare the dining table and to select the cutlery, crockery and condiments from the usual cupboards or drawers.
- Encourage Ken to clear away afterwards.

QCS PAL ACTIVITY PROFILE

SENSORY ACTIVITY LEVEL OF ABILITY

Name: Millie Dunbar

Date: 1 September 2022

Likely abilities

- Is likely to be responding to bodily sensations. Can be guided to carry out single-step activities
- Can carry out more complex activities if they are broken down into one step at a time

Likely limitations

- May not have any conscious plan to carry out a movement to achieve a particular end result
- May be relying on others to make social contact

Caregiver's role

- To enable the person to experience the effect of the activity on their senses
- To break the activity into one step at a time
- To keep directions simple and understandable
- To approach and make the first contact with the person

Using the PAL Activity Profile to support the person

Position of objects	Ensure that the person becomes aware of objects and materials by making bodily contact.
Verbal directions	Limit requests to carry out actions to the naming of the action and of the object involved, e.g. 'lift your arm', 'hold the brush'.
Demonstrated directions	Demonstrate to the person the action on the object. Break the activity down into one step at a time.
Working with others	Others must approach the person and make the first contact. Use touch and the person's name to sustain the social contact.
Activity characteristics	The activity is used as an opportunity for a sensory experience. This may be multisensory. Repetitive actions are appropriate.

Suitable leisure activities

- Identify an activity of interest to the person based on knowledge of their interests, career, home life and so on, or select one of the activities suggested below as a starting point.
    - Sensory box, smells, food tasting, hand massage, exercises, music and singing, dancing, sweeping, polishing, wiping tables, etc.

Activity plan:

One-to-one sensory activities – hand massage, sensory box

One-to-one single-step activities – wool winding, laundry folding

As Millie is engaging in activities at a sensory level, collection of further information about her specific preferences will enable care givers to support her to enjoy the sensory experience of each of her preferred objects. This will support a truly person-centred approach that can be tailored to Millie by using the PAL Individual Action Plan.

QCS PAL INDIVIDUAL ACTION PLAN

Name: Millie Dunbar

Date: 1 September 2022

DRESSING
Favourite garments
Skirts and jumpers

Preferred routine
Has breakfast in her dressing gown and then has a wash and gets dressed

Grooming likes and dislikes
Doesn't wear make-up or nail varnish. Doesn't use soap on her face, only water

Method

- Encourage discussion about the clothing to be worn for the day: is it suitable for the weather or the occasion? Is it a favourite item?
- Spend time colour-matching items of clothing and select accessories.
- Break down the activity into manageable chunks: help lay the clothes out in order so that underclothing is at the top of the pile. If Millie wishes to be helped, talk her through the task: 'Put on your underclothes', 'Now put on your skirt and blouse.'
- Encourage Millie to check her appearance in the mirror.

BATHING/SHOWERING
Favourite toiletries
Imperial Leather soap

Preferred routine
Wash in the morning and bath in the evening

Bathing likes and dislikes
Loves bubble bath, prefers small towels

Method

- Break down the activity into manageable chunks: suggest that Millie fills the bath. When that is accomplished, suggest that she gathers together items such as soap, shampoo, flannel and towels.
- When Millie is in the bath suggest that she soaps and rinses her upper body. When that is accomplished, suggest that she soaps and rinses her lower body.
- Ensure that bathing items are on view and that containers are clearly labelled.

- Have attractive objects around the bathroom such as unusual bath oil bottles or shells and encourage discussion and exploration of them.

DINING

Favourite foods

Full English breakfast with fried eggs. Chocolate

Preferred routine

Needs to sit facing the window so that she can leave the table easily

Dining likes and dislikes

None known

Method

- Store cutlery and crockery in view and encourage Millie to select own tools for dining.
- Offer food using simple choices.
- Create a social atmosphere using table decorations and music, and promote conversation.

Chapter 9

IMPLEMENTING INTERVENTIONS

ACTIVITIES

When considering the range of activities in which we engage, it may be helpful to split them into three main categories: personal care tasks, domestic tasks, such as cleaning, cooking and gardening, and leisure interests. In addition, considering the sensory needs and preferences of all individuals, but particularly those at a sensory or a reflex activity level of ability, can lead to specialist interventions using sensory activities. These are explored in depth in the next chapter, 'Planning and Implementing Sensory Interventions', which has been contributed by sensory preferences specialist Professor Lesley Collier.

A person with cognitive impairment can be helped to carry out any activities using the PAL Activity Profile, and the Individual Action Plan pays particular attention to the personal care activities.

Most caregivers find that there is insufficient time for the person they care for to carry out all activities at their own level of ability, particularly when the pace of the person is slowed. For many family caregivers, the demands of enabling the person they care for to work through the steps of an activity can be physically and emotionally exhausting. Attempting to work to one's full potential in all areas of daily life will be equally exhausting to the person with cognitive impairment. For caregivers in communal settings, such as residential homes or hospitals, there are often not enough staff to allow this amount of individual time with people.

The solution is to give priority to the activities that have the most importance for the person with cognitive impairment, so that they are able to do as much as is possible in those aspects, while helping them to conserve energy by giving increased assistance in areas that are felt to be of lesser importance. For example, Elsie, who has always paid a lot of attention to her physical appearance, may be enabled to carry out grooming tasks to her full potential, but the domestic chores such as making the bed can be done for her. George, who shows great enthusiasm for the social and the dining aspects of mealtimes and has begun to respond to the sensory experiences around him, may prefer to accept assistance with his bathing and dressing needs, so that he has more time and energy to enjoy engaging with others through these sensory opportunities.

Caregivers who are close relatives or friends will have a wealth of information about the life history and the personality of the person with cognitive impairment. The PAL Life History Profile (see Chapter 6) is a useful guide to the gathering and recording of this type of information and a valuable starting point in planning which occupations will be of most interest. If the person is living in a communal setting, the caregiver can share this information with the whole team, including the activity providers and volunteers, and, with the person's permission, with their visitors so that the most appropriate occupations are offered. If the person lives at home with a caregiver, and services such as home care are provided, this information can be also shared with those service providers.

Caregivers sometimes feel that it is inappropriate to encourage the person with cognitive impairment to carry out an occupation that cannot be performed at as high a standard as it was previously. If the person is still interested in the activity, it is likely that they will still enjoy the opportunity to carry it out and, if the person is concerned about the standard of the final outcome, by presenting the activity using the guidelines in the PAL Activity Profile, the person will be able to engage with the activity in manageable stages. For many people with cognitive impairment, it is not the final end product that is so important, but the opportunity to engage in the process of doing the activity. When caregivers recognize this they can place less emphasis on what has been achieved in terms of final product and more emphasis on what has been achieved in terms of experiencing the activity.

The knowledge of a person's interests and familiar routines, together with an understanding of how they best carry out activities, can be utilized to ensure that the occupations which are engaged in are unique to the individual. As the person is provided with opportunities to become meaningfully occupied, it may well be that their cognitive and functional ability will improve. By adopting a facilitating approach, the person's level of ability should be sustained for longer. Even when a person's ability level decreases, as is possible given the nature of some of the conditions causing cognitive impairment, it is unlikely that their interests will change. Therefore these may continue, using the PAL Activity Profile for the new level. For example, John may be helped to engage in gardening activities using the Activity Profile at a *planned* activity level of ability. In the future, he may lose some of these abilities and it may become appropriate still to present gardening opportunities to him, but use the PAL Activity Profile for an *exploratory* activity level of ability that will give guidance on how to continue to facilitate his gardening interest. As his condition progresses and he moves to a *sensory* and then to a *reflex* level of ability, the PAL Profile will guide individuals in how to support ongoing engagement in this activity that has personal meaning to John. They will also be encouraged to use therapeutic interactions so that the activity becomes more concerned with 'being' than with 'doing': this is an important part of personhood, where the sense of being is provided through these meaningful interactions and connections with another.

It is proposed that it is possible to take any activity in which a person is interested, and use the appropriate PAL Activity Profile to present it at the right level for that individual. Examples of some typical activities, which can be presented at either a *planned*, *exploratory*, *sensory* or *reflex* activity level, are presented on the next pages. These are intended to give a flavour of how the information in the PAL Activity Profile can be translated into everyday practice.

To assist carers to facilitate further leisure activities, Part 2 of this guide includes ideas for four activity packs. Several possible activities are described, with sources for obtaining them and guidance for carrying them out with individuals who have different levels of ability as revealed by the completion of the PAL Instrument Checklist.

ACTIVITY: GARDENING

PLANNED ACTIVITY LEVEL

- Plan a planting task by looking through seed catalogues, gardening magazines or visiting a garden centre.
- Encourage the person to take charge of getting objects off the gardening shelf/ trolley, and of planting the plants out in the garden or a tub.
- Hand over the responsibility for watering or weeding (the person may need reminding).
- Encourage the person to clean up after the task is completed and to put away tools in the appropriate places.

EXPLORATORY ACTIVITY LEVEL

- Encourage the person to be creative with the planting arrangement, select unusual containers and spend time discussing what plants will look attractive in them.
- Arrange a workspace close to where the objects are on view. Ensure that items are obvious: keep plant labels and the potting compost bag turned towards the person so that the writing and pictures are visible.
- Break down the task into manageable chunks: suggest to the person that they use a trowel or old spoon to fill the tray or bowl with potting compost; when that is accomplished, suggest that the plants be placed in the container; and when that is achieved, suggest that the person fills a watering can and waters the plants.
- Create a social occasion, perhaps use the activity as an opportunity to reminisce about previous gardens or to discuss favourite plants.

SENSORY ACTIVITY LEVEL

- Prepare a table with the planting equipment.
- Encourage the person to use their hands to put the potting compost into the containers. Spend time crumbling it and smoothing it with the fingers.
- Plant scented herbs or lemon-scented geraniums. Encourage the person to crush a little in their fingers and to smell or taste them.
- Enter 'watering' into the person's weekly planner or diary and accompany them on this task.

REFLEX ACTIVITY LEVEL

- Position the person next to you when you carry out the planting task. Ensure that they are comfortable and can see what you are doing.
- Keep equipment that is not being used out of the person's line of vision.

✓

- Offer a plant to the person to smell by placing your fingers over theirs and, together, gently crush the plant. Raise the person's hand to their face and suggest that they 'smell' the plant.
- Use your body language of smiling and nodding to reinforce that this is a pleasant experience for you too.

ACTIVITY: PREPARING A FRUIT SALAD

PLANNED ACTIVITY LEVEL

- Use a recipe card with a picture of the end result.
- Encourage the person to follow the directions on the recipe card to make the fruit juice base for the salad.
- Encourage the person to take charge of cutting the fruit up and arranging it in the bowl.

EXPLORATORY ACTIVITY LEVEL

- Use a tin of fruit as a base for the salad so that the juice does not have to be made. Add fresh orange juice to it so that there is sufficient juice. Have a selection of fresh fruit to add to the base.
- Arrange a workplace close to where the equipment is on view. Ensure that items needed are obvious: keep the tin of fruit and the orange juice container turned so that the labels are visible.
- Encourage the person to be creative about selecting the fruit and the container to be used, and spend time discussing which colours of fruit will look attractive.
- Break down the task into manageable chunks: suggest to the person that they open the tin and empties it into the salad container; when that is accomplished suggest that you will peel the fruit while the person chops it.
- Create a social occasion out of the task, use it as an opportunity to reminisce about family meals or to discuss favourite foods.

SENSORY ACTIVITY LEVEL

- Prepare the table with an orange, apple, pear and seedless grapes, a container and the cutlery. Open a tin of pineapple to act as a base for the salad.
- Encourage the person to handle each piece of fruit, to feel the texture of the skin and to smell it.
- Break down the task into one step at a time: peel the orange and suggest that the person splits the segments while you chop the apple and pear. When this is accomplished, suggest to the person that they pick the grapes off the stem and put them into the container with the rest of the salad.
- When finished, encourage the person to smell and to lick their fingers and to enjoy the aroma and the look of the fruit salad.

REFLEX ACTIVITY LEVEL

- Position the person next to you when you prepare the fruit salad. Ensure that the person is comfortable and can see what you are doing.

✓

- Only have on view the piece of fruit which you are preparing; keep the fruit and objects that are not in immediate use out of the person's line of vision.
- Place a piece of soft fruit, such as a banana or kiwi fruit, in the person's hand and assist them to hold it by placing your fingers over theirs. Raise the person's hand to their face and encourage them to smell and taste the fruit.
- Use your body language of smiling and nodding to reinforce that this is a pleasant experience for you too.

Chapter 10

PLANNING AND IMPLEMENTING SENSORY INTERVENTIONS

Lesley Collier

INTRODUCTION

Activity for people with dementia has long been considered to be an important aspect in maintaining well-being; however, there is growing consensus that activities and occupations for people with moderate to severe dementia are either not available or fail to match their abilities and skill levels. Sensory activity may be a way of engaging people with more severe cognitive impairment. This chapter will explore the role of sensation and activity for people with severe cognitive impairment and suggests how sensory activity and multisensory environments can be implemented using the PAL Activity Profile.

THE ROLE OF ACTIVITY AND OCCUPATION IN COGNITIVE DECLINE

Identifying suitable activity for people with dementia appears to be guided by the assumption that an increase in activity is positively correlated with an increased sense of well-being. However, much debate remains regarding the most suitable type of activities to use for people with moderate to severe dementia, the difficulty in assessing well-being among this client group and the anatomical impact of taking part in an activity. Given that people with moderate to severe dementia may not be able to participate in hobbies enjoyed in the past, it may be the components of that activity that need to be presented or even the sensory features. For example, a woman who enjoyed baking may experience pleasure being able to knead dough and being able to taste the finished product, despite not being able to complete the activity as a whole. Identifying these components may be critical in constructing a sensory activity that is suitable and desirable for the person. This form of activity may also provide a level of stimulation that increases levels of arousal and attention, which in turn may have a positive impact on the person's ability to participate. The theory bases underpinning the level of stimulation needed to facilitate participation in activity for people with moderate to severe cognitive decline will be explored later. Prior to this, consideration will be given to the sensory impairments older people may have which influence their ability to process sensory information, the impact of these sensory changes on activity, and the subsequent potential of sensory stimulation for neurogenesis.

SENSORY CHANGES AND SENSORY DEPRIVATION, AND THEIR IMPACT ON ACTIVITY

Sensory deprivation is a phenomenon where stimulation to an individual's senses is greatly reduced. Common characteristics of sensory deprivation include disorientation, irritability, confusion, lethargy and hallucinatory phenomena (Zubek 1969). These are features that are also common in dementia, among other neurological conditions. Therefore, by addressing these features of sensory deprivation with sensory stimulation it may be possible to reduce some of the characteristics of dementia. Sensory deprivation can be exacerbated by admission to residential accommodation or hospital (Voelkl, Ellis and Walker 2003), and drugs such as neuroleptics, with their associated side effects such as sedation, only further reduce opportunities for sensory stimulation (Burns *et al.* 2002).

This is supported by empirical evidence that older people with dementia are at increased risk of sensory deprivation due to sensory changes, deterioration of cognitive skills (loss of social skills and executive functioning) and environmental restrictions such as residential care or living alone (Bower 1967; MacDonald 2002; Norberg, Melin and Asplund 1986). Sensory changes can be experienced through sensory alterations associated with ageing: specifically visual changes, hearing loss and loss of taste and smell (Appollonio *et al.* 1996; Zegeer 1986). For example, Weale (1963) estimates that the eye of a 60-year-old person receives only a third of light through the pupil compared to that of a 20-year-old person. Consequently, a stronger light stimulus is needed to achieve the same effect. As vision, hearing, taste and smell are critical for social interaction as well as learning and orientation to the environment, a loss of these senses may lead to dependency, reduced quality of life and isolation (Valentijn *et al.* 2005; Zegeer 1986). Stronger stimuli, greater contrast between stimuli and allowing time to process the stimuli (as sensory processing takes longer in the older person) can offset the effect of sensory changes (Laurienti *et al.* 2006). This may maximize the person's remaining sensory abilities (Heyn 2003). However, given variation in stimulus intensity and age-related decline, it is difficult to know what constitutes stimulus effectiveness. Very few studies have explored the relationship between sensory processing and selection of appropriate stimulation or even which senses are the most appropriate to stimulate (Corso 1971; Keller *et al.* 1999; Laurienti *et al.* 2006). Brown *et al.* (2001) go some way to identifying the preferred mode of stimulation, but even their method of assessment is open to interpretation.

As well as considering the need for sensory stimulation, consideration needs also to be given to the complexity of the stimulation (uni-sensory stimulation versus multisensory stimulation). Research suggests that multisensory stimulation is preferable to uni-sensory stimulation (Hairston *et al.* 2003), although the number of stimuli needed to achieve a suitable multisensory experience is unclear. Laurienti *et al.* (2006) suggest that this is dependent on the level of deterioration of sensory processing in older people, but increased numbers of sensory modalities are more beneficial when the sensory signal is ambiguous. While Laurienti *et al.*'s study used 'well' older people, this finding would also appear to be relevant to older people with dementia, where the majority of stimulation may be perceived to be ambiguous due to limited cognitive ability. Therefore, assessment of preferred sensory modality and activity characteristics would appear to be paramount in selecting the most appropriate level of sensory stimulation within an activity. By getting the level and intensity of stimulation right there may be a potential to influence neural reorganization (neurogenesis).

NEUROGENESIS IN THE AGEING BRAIN AND ITS IMPACT ON ACTIVITY

In addition to positive effects of engaging in activity on cognition and behaviour, evidence from neurogenesis studies show that activity also has a positive effect on the development of the brain. Neurogenesis is the proliferation, survival, migration and differentiation of neural cells (Lomassese *et al.* 2000). Early studies (Bennett, Rosenzweig and Diamond 1969; Hebb 1949) identified that sensory enrichment has an effect on neural development as demonstrated by increased brain weight, cortical thickness and increased synaptogenesis (creation of new synapses). Later studies have revealed how both young and old brains have a remarkable capacity to be shaped by environmental input (Bavelier and Neville 2002; Kobayashi, Ohashi and Ando 2002). Evidence also exists to support the theory that behavioural and environmental factors can influence neurogenesis (Kempermann, Gast and Gage 2002; Rochefort *et al.* 2002). Indeed, the rate of neural proliferation appears to be highly sensitive to environmental factors and social interaction (Sandeman and Sandeman 2000). This has implications for people with cognitive decline, as activity and, what is also important, an enriched environment may have an effect on the progression of the disease process.

In the adult, neurogenesis has been identified in two key areas of the brain: the olfactory bulb and its associated areas, and the dentate gyrus of the hippocampus. The dentate gyrus (part of the hippocampus, a temporal lobe structure) is known to have a pivotal role in higher cortical functions such as memory and learning. This theory is underpinned by many animal studies which highlight the benefit of physical exercise, social interaction and environmental enrichment on the neural plasticity and brain weight of rats (Coq and Xerri 2001; Rochefort *et al.* 2002; Sandeman and Sandeman 2000). Rats that were exposed to environmental enrichment showed an increase in brain weight; moreover, those reared in complex environments, during ageing, performed better on learning and memory tasks (Coq and Xerri 2001). Experiments with mice also revealed an improvement in short-term memory among those exposed to enriched environments. It is thought that this enriched experience allows the animal to adapt to their changing environment (Lomassese *et al.* 2000; Rochefort *et al.* 2002). These findings have also been replicated in studies with crayfish and crickets, where enrichment with sensory stimuli (visual, olfactory, auditory and tactile) increased the production of neural growth and triggered motor activity and exploration (Lomassese *et al.* 2000).

One of the challenges in stimulating neurogenic effects in the ageing brain might be related to the difficulties of somatic stimulation, where ageing impairs sensory functions such as tactile sensitivity, sensory motor coordination, locomotion and exploratory activities (Coq and Xerri 2001). Decreased sensory function and stress are two features that are common in dementia, and severe stress is also known to decrease adult hippocampal neurogenesis (Kempermann *et al.* 2002). This reduction of neurogenic regulation has been linked to hippocampal pathology, including Alzheimer's disease (Kempermann *et al.* 2002). This diminished regulation may help explain aspects of cognitive decline seen in dementia (Kempermann *et al.* 2002; McKhann 2002). As studies indicate neurogenesis occurs in the hippocampal dentate gyrus throughout life, with low baseline levels only evident in later life, it seems appropriate that activity and environmental enrichment should be maintained in old age (Kobayashi *et al.* 2002). Indeed, Kempermann *et al.* (2002) noted that continued exposure to a challenging, stimulating environment has the potential to invoke a large upregulation of neural plasticity, regardless of age, and even after environmental stimulation is discontinued the presence of neurogenesis can still be detected, suggesting that regular stimulation has a carry-over effect. Arendt (2001) also reported that behavioural experience not only organizes sensory cortical representation but also the rate of neurogenesis in the hippocampus, suggesting regular stimulation may enhance neurogenesis. It also appears the novelty of sensory stimuli rather than continual enriched stimuli affects adult hippocampal neurogenesis (Lomassese *et al.* 2000). This is evident in environments where the television is left constantly switched on and no one watches it, in comparison to an unexpected visitor who draws attention. Although our understanding of neurogenesis in humans is limited, these animal studies support the notion that regular activity and a stimulating environment have beneficial effects on cognitive functioning, and, despite the ageing process, the hippocampus maintains the potential for neurogenesis. It would also appear that the novelty of stimuli is important in leading to a change in neural structure (Lomassese *et al.* 2000; Lu and Zhao 2005); therefore, activity should be adaptable in order to maintain interest through novelty and variety of stimuli offered.

Activity for people with moderate to severe dementia is clearly important; however, the key issues revolve around the selection of suitable activity which matches the specific needs of this group. Underpinning this are several theory bases, not normally applied in dementia, which may assist in the facilitation of sensory activity. These will be considered as a justification for a suitable activity alongside a summary of the desirable features of activity for people with cognitive decline.

The key theories influencing the facilitation of sensory activity can be roughly divided into those relating to the individual and those relating to the environment in which the activity takes place. The use of the PAL tool influences the approach adopted by the caregiver in facilitating and enabling activity. The use of the PAL tool to support caregivers will be described later in this chapter.

THE INFLUENCE OF INDIVIDUAL CHARACTERISTICS ON PARTICIPATION IN ACTIVITY: THE MODEL OF SENSORY PROCESSING

The problem of sensory deprivation may be exacerbated by the older person failing to process sensory information, due to cerebral atrophy. Dunn's Sensory Processing Model, originally developed with children (Dunn 2001), has been expanded to include adults (Brown and Dunn 2002) and explains behavioural responses to sensation. The model suggests that people fall within one of four sensory quadrants: low registration, sensory seeking, sensory sensitivity and sensory avoidance. The sensory quadrant in which an individual falls determines the types of responding strategies they may exhibit (Table 10.1).

Table 10.1: Dunn's Model of Sensory Processing (Brown and Dunn 2002)

Threshold/Reactivity	Responding strategies	
	Passive – behaves passively	Active – aware of threshold, endeavours to control sensory input
High threshold with low reactivity – needs a lot of stimulus to reach the threshold (tendency to be unresponsive or needs more intensive sensory stimuli)	Low-registration quadrant Does not notice sensory events in everyday life or is slow to respond 'I don't smell things that other people smell' 'I don't get jokes very quickly'	Sensory-seeking quadrant Looks for sensory experiences in everyday life 'I like spicy food' 'I enjoy having my hair cut'

Low threshold with high reactivity – does not need much stimulus to reach threshold (tendency to be overly responsive or annoyed with sensory stimuli)	Sensory-sensitivity quadrant Readily notices sensory stimuli and may be uncomfortable or distracted by them 'I don't like heights' 'I don't like messy rooms'	Sensory-avoiding quadrant Deliberately acts to reduce or prevent exposure to sensory stimuli 'I only eat familiar food' 'I always wear gloves during messy activities'

Thresholds indicate how much stimulation is needed before the person responds. The responding strategies reflect an active response, whereby an effort is made to seek out or avoid stimuli; or a passive response, whereby little or no effort is made to respond to stimuli. People with a high threshold and passive responding strategies fall within the low-registration quadrant. They do not notice sensory events in daily life that others notice readily, for example having dirty hands. Individuals with high thresholds and active responding strategies fall within the sensory-seeking quadrant. They enjoy sensory experiences and will actively seek them out; examples include people who like fairground rides. Those with low thresholds and passive responding strategies fall within the sensory-sensitivity quadrant. They notice sensory events more readily than others and are easily distracted; for example, they notice changes in temperature or changes in a familiar environment. Those with low thresholds and active responding strategies fall within the sensory-avoidance quadrant. They find ways to avoid sensory input during the day; examples include leaving a noisy environment or creating rituals, as seen in those on the autism spectrum (Brown *et al.* 2001).

This model may explain the responses of people with dementia to sensory stimuli. For example, someone constantly playing with a petticoat may be demonstrating the behaviours of a sensory seeker; those who dislike being touched may be demonstrating the behaviours of a sensory avoider. Although the model describes four distinct quadrants, it is possible for individuals to fall across quadrants. For example, a person may display elements of sensory sensitivity and sensory avoidance by readily noticing things they dislike and actively avoiding them. The model offers little explanation of how a person straddling two or more quadrants may be engaged in activity, but may help to explain why some activities fail to engage the person.

However, the Model of Sensory Processing does account for the nervous system's threshold for acting and the person's propensity for responding to those thresholds (Dunn and Westman 1997). The model suggests that our personal neurological threshold (the point at which we respond or react) causes us to respond in a certain way (behaviour). Dunn suggests that our thresholds are on a continuum and have the potential to fluctuate in different circumstances. However, there is still debate over whether our neurological threshold is a trait or a state characteristic that can fluctuate in different conditions (Dunn and Brown 1997; Pohl, Dunn and Brown 2003).

Given that Dunn suggests that we all respond differently to sensory stimuli, then sensory activity should arguably be tailored to meet individual needs. These needs may also change with age. Indeed, Pohl *et al.*'s (2003) study explored whether there are age-related differences in sensory processing using Dunn's Adult Sensory Profile (Brown and Dunn 2002). The Adult Sensory Profile is a questionnaire-based assessment developed from the Model of Sensory Processing. The profile uses responses to everyday sensory experiences to identify sensory preferences (Brown and Dunn 2002). The results reveal that there are significant differences in the way older adults (65 years +) and young to middle-aged adults (19–64 years) notice sensory stimuli. In particular, older adults notice and seek out fewer stimuli than those less than 65 years of age. This behaviour is possibly exacerbated in dementia, as the person with dementia has to allocate more attentional resources to perceive and interpret sensory information (Baddeley *et al.* 2001; Perry and Hodges 1999). This behaviour is also likely to exacerbate the risk of sensory deprivation as there may be fewer resources left for other cognitively demanding tasks. This illustrates the need to enhance the sensory component of activity, in order to assist with the perception and interpretation of sensory information.

That individuals have different sensory needs may contribute to understanding why many people with dementia fail to participate successfully in activity. Unlike 'well' older people, they may be unable to modify their interaction with the sensory activity in order to adjust the level of stimulation. Thus, an understanding of which sensory quadrant an individual falls within may assist with the selection of appropriately stimulating activities. For example, a person who is a sensory seeker may require activities that provide more intense stimulation, such as getting their hands into clay. In contrast, a sensory avoider may find some activities uncomfortable if the sensory demands are too great, such as being part of a large group. Sensory processing is also reliant on the individual being able to integrate the sensory information. Ayres's Theory of Sensory Integration embraces many of the premises of sensory process and, despite being based on work with children with developmental delay, may also go some way to explain why people with cognitive impairment have problems with processing the sensory components of activity.

THE INFLUENCE OF INDIVIDUAL CHARACTERISTICS ON PARTICIPATION IN ACTIVITY: SENSORY INTEGRATION THEORY

Ayres developed Sensory Integration (SI) Theory to explain the relationship between sensory processing and behavioural responses when they cannot be attributed to neurological damage alone. Ayres (1979) reflects that the ability to cope with the environment diminishes in the absence of an adequate level of stimulus. Once in a state of deprivation, the person's environmental coping process becomes dysfunctional and responses to sensory input become maladaptive. SI Theory was developed to explain the relationship between behaviour and neural functioning. Ayres defined the sensory integrative process as the ability to organize sensory information for use (Ayres 1979), and expanded it by saying 'the brain must select, enhance, inhibit, compare and associate the sensory information in a flexible, constant changing pattern...the brain must integrate it' (p.11). SI Theory suggests that opportunities for engagement in sensorimotor activities rich in tactile, vestibular and proprioceptive sensations will facilitate sensory integration (Schaaf and Miller 2005). This approach must accompany the 'just right challenge'. This challenge is to provide an activity that is achievable, age-appropriate and goal-directed. Active engagement in the challenge will ensure that abilities are practised, rehearsed and retained. King (1983) utilized these principles for people with schizophrenia to address performance deficits in cognition, communication, affect, praxis and activity level. She found an improvement in praxis as well as communication, which led her to conclude that gross motor activities such as those used in SI go some way to improve 'psychiatric status' (King 1983). However, King did acknowledge that these improvements were not sustained and research in this area lacked methodological rigour. Using SI principles in this way with adults rather than children led to an alternative approach to address the maladaptive responses of older people with dementia (Ross and Burdick 1981).

An evaluation of the SI approach was carried out by Corcoran and Barrett (1987) among older people with dementia in residential care. Results revealed substantial clinical improvement in the experimental group in terms of automatic postural correction and increased attention, and significant improvement in communication and task performance scores. Although this study supports the use of SI with older people with dementia, it is limited by its small sample size. Subsequent studies in this area are also limited, with the majority concentrating on children with developmental delay (Roley *et al.* 2003; Smith *et al.* 2005).

Although individual characteristics are paramount in selecting appropriate activity, performance components of activity must be considered as well. The Model of Sensory Integration highlights the relationship between matching individual ability, task complexity and environmental demands. Dunn (2001), Ayres (1979) and Corcoran and Barrett (1987) all emphasize the relationship between the person's ability to process and integrate sensory information and the impact of the environment on this process. So often attention is paid to the activity but not to the environment in which it takes place. This environmental influence will be explored through the model of sensoristasis and environmental domicility.

THE ENVIRONMENTAL INFLUENCE ON ACTIVITY: SENSORISTASIS

The environmental demands on people with severe dementia have been explored using the Progressively Lowered Stress Threshold (PLST) model (Hall and Buckwalter 1987) and Lawton's ecological model (Lawton 1986). These models suggest that if environmental press (sensory demand) exceeds the individual's ability to process sensory information then function and behaviour will be negatively affected (Kovach 2000). They propose a delicate balance between the environment and the individual. However, the models offer no explanation of how this balance may be achieved. Kovach (2000) expanded the PLST model to explore balance and named this 'sensoristasis'. Kovach suggests that optimal functional performance will occur if there is a balance of sensory calming and sensory-stimulating activities. An imbalance in sensoristasis may lead to functional and behavioural problems (Figure 10.1).

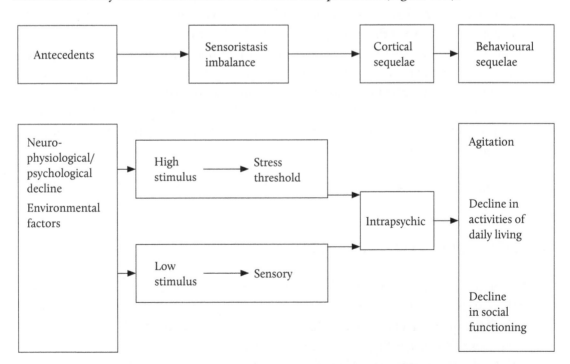

Figure 10.1: Model of imbalances in sensoristasis as applied to people with dementia (adapted from Kovach 2000)

Tenets of the model include:

- People with severe dementia experience imbalance of sensoristasis, caused by neuro-physiological or environmental factors such as a noisy living area or busy shop.
- Too much high-stimulus activity (noisy environment) can result in one's stress threshold being exceeded. This will occur at a lower stress threshold if the activity is unpleasant or the person is required to process too much sensory information at a pace that is too rapid for them. An example may be where a person is encouraged to attend a large party with unfamiliar people.
- Too low a level of stimulus can create a state of sensory deprivation. A common example of induced deprivation is where a carer or healthcare professional does so much for the person that their level of activity is substantially decreased.
- States of exceeded stress threshold or sensory deprivation can lead to intrapsychic discomfort (agitated behaviour, decline in activities of daily living and social skills).

By pacing activities to provide a balance between sensory calming and sensory-stimulating activity, sensoristasis may be achieved.

Kovach applied this model to people with severe dementia and found that, as the dementia progressed, people needed longer periods of sensory-calming activities between sensory-stimulating activities in order to maximize periods of engagement in activity (Kovach and Meyer Arnold 1997). She also found that stimulating multiple senses (sight, sound, touch, taste and smell) was associated with longer periods of engagement in activity for people with late-stage dementia (Kovach and Magliocco 1998). This supports the notion that multisensory activity may be more engaging for people with moderate to severe dementia than uni-sensory activity.

Voelkl (1990) used the tenets of Lawton's ecological model to conduct focus groups with nursing staff, in order to identify environmental barriers to engagement in activity. This model describes the balance between environmental and social demands (Lawton 1986). The results highlighted the problems of attending to different environmental needs due to the physical environment, but also of the management of staff attitudes of how time should be spent. More specifically, staff felt that their time was taken up in nursing duties rather than facilitating activity and residents had low expectation of activity taking place. Many activities offered to people with dementia fail to address environmental demands, being conducted in noisy environments often with limited numbers of staff. Consequently, although the activity may be of a suitable level, the person may fail to engage in the activity due to competing demands from the environment.

The balance between environmental demands and activity was also explored by Csikszentmihalyi in his work on flow.

ACTIVITY CHARACTERISTICS: FLOW

Csikszentmihalyi's work (1975) provides an interesting focus on activity and well-being. In particular, he describes the need for balance between the challenge of the activity and the skills of the individual needed in order to attain engagement or 'flow'.

Flow is described as the sense of total involvement in an activity driven by self-directed goals (Csikszentmihalyi 1975). Flow illustrates the proposed relationship between the skills of the individual and the challenge offered by the activity (Csikszentmihalyi 1975). The experience of the activity is perceived to be most positive (flow) when the individual believes that the activity or environment contains sufficient opportunities (challenges) which are matched to their personal ability (skill level). If the balance is right, a sense of well-being can be achieved (Csikszentmihalyi and LeFevre 1989). Many of the activities offered to people with dementia would appear not to address the issues of skill level and challenge, which may be an explanation for some of the apathetic or agitated behaviours demonstrated by some people with dementia. These behaviours suggest lack of engagement or loss of a state of flow.

The concept of flow has been explored with well adults (Jacobs 1994). This study reports that participants felt at their best when flow conditions were present (suitable challenges and in control). Participants described flow experiences as including such moods as 'being happy', 'involved', 'positive' and 'productive' (Jacobs 1994). Although no such studies have been carried out for people with dementia, the principles of flow have the potential to be achieved if the environment and activity are well matched. By using the PAL tool, the caregiver is also able to match their facilitation skills to the ability level of the person. There appears to be no reason why, by finding activities via the Personal History Profile that are intrinsically motivating, presenting and supporting the person with the right level of facilitation skills as indicated by the PAL Activity Profile, that a sense of flow should not be achieved by a person with dementia. This improved engagement could, in turn, promote a sense of well-being (Emerson 1998).

In summary, three key areas support the use of activity with older people with dementia. First, activity has the potential positively to influence cognition and physical health. Evidence also supports the counterargument that poor cognition leads to reductions in activity. Second, reductions in activity lead to a reduced sense of well-being, quality of life and functional ability; however, these reductions are reversible given the facilitation of suitable activity. Third, animal studies support the idea that activity increases the proliferation of brain cells that are important for memory and learning. Without this level of stimulation, sensory deprivation may occur, leading to deterioration of cognitive skills. Therefore, sensory deprivation may be an important determinant of activity. Taken together, this evidence suggests that engaging in an activity that is highly stimulating, novel and of suitable complexity is likely to benefit people with cognitive impairment.

The theories described above offer a framework from which a suitable sensory activity can be selected and initiated. They all suggest that the activity should include an appropriate level of stimulation that challenges the individual to reach their maximum potential (sensory stimulation versus sensory deprivation). The activity should be designed to address individual sensory needs, such as offering a stronger stimulus if initial attempts are unnoticed (sensory processing), and be offered alongside familiar activities and routines (sensory integration). The activity should occur on a regular basis and offer a 'just-right challenge' as the person with dementia will find it easier to cope with the demands of the environment if adequate stimulation is provided (sensory integration). The levels or intensity of the activity may need to be adjusted depending on individual needs. Sensoristasis and flow both explore the relationship between individual competency and environmental demand. If there is an imbalance between the level of environmental stimulation and the person's ability to process that information, the activity will fail. Finally, if the complexity of the activity, individual needs and environmental demands are matched, engagement may be achieved.

SENSORY ACTIVITY AND MULTISENSORY ENVIRONMENTS

Multisensory environments or sensory activities are designed to stimulate the primary senses of touch, taste, sight, sound, smell and movement without the need for intellectual activity.

Engagement with the sensory components of the activity is encouraged via non-directive approaches. The essence of a sensory environment is to allow people the time, space and opportunity to enjoy the environment at their own pace, free from unrealistic expectations of others.

Sensory environments usually include objects to stimulate all the senses and are best viewed as a 'tool box' from which specific objects can be selected to provide stimulation for the person. The multisensory 'tool box' should include a range of objects to stimulate:

- Sight – for example, optic fibres, bubble tubes, coloured fabric, coloured lights.
- Sound – music based on the person's preference. Music that is upbeat will be more stimulating than slow melodic music. Alternatively, bird song, sounds of the sea or whale song could be used.
- Touch – for example, vibrating cushions, textured fabric, optic fibres.
- Taste – to stimulate taste rather than to feed, so examples might include sherbet, peppermint or orange, or textures such as jelly, honey or popping chocolate.
- Smell – for example, familiar aromas such as cut grass, lavender or lemon, or aromatic smells such as perfume.
- Movement – proprioceptive and vestibular stimulation, for example rocking chairs, wobble boards, positioning on equipment to encourage reach beyond the midline.

Sensory objects should be selected based on the person's sensory preferences. These can be identified by carrying out a standardized sensory assessment such as the Adult Sensory Profile (Brown and Dunn 2002) or the Sensory Assessment and Profiling Tool (Collier 2005). Alternatively, a sensory assessment can be carried out by observing sensory responses to everyday sensory activities, and activities in which people enjoy engaging with; for example, a person who enjoys gardening, baking and dress making would appear to enjoy activities that have a strong tactile (touch) element. A person who takes regular walks and enjoys dancing would be a person who might prefer a sensory activity with a strong movement (proprioceptive) approach.

Using the QCS PAL Instrument to create the Activity Profile and your understanding of a person's sensory preference based on their Life History Profile, a sensory activity can be constructed to meet individual needs. The relevant PAL Activity Profile for multisensory environments can be found in Chapter 1.

REFERENCES

Appollonio, I., Carabellese, C., Frattola, L. and Trabucchi, M. (1996) 'Effects of sensory aids on the quality of life and mortality of elderly people: A multivariate analysis.' *Age and Ageing*, 25(2), 89–96.

Arendt, T. (2001) 'Alzheimer's disease as a disorder of mechanisms underlying structural brain organisation.' *Neuroscience*, 102(4), 723–765.

Ayres, A. (1979) *Sensory Integration and the Child*. Los Angeles, CA: Western Psychological Services.

Baddeley, A., Baddeley, H., Bucks, R. and Wilcock, G. (2001) 'Attentional control in Alzheimer's disease.' *Brain*, 124(8), 1492–1508.

Bavelier, D. and Neville, H. (2002) 'Cross-modal plasticity: Where and how?' *Nature Reviews Neuroscience*, 3(6), 443–452.

Bennett, E., Rosenzweig, M. and Diamond, M. (1969) 'Rat brain: Effects of environmental enhancement on wet and dry weights.' *Science*, 163(3869), 825–826.

Bower, H. (1967) 'Sensory stimulation and the treatment of senile dementia.' *The Medical Journal of Australia*, 22(1), 1113–1119.

Brown, C. and Dunn, W. (2002) *Adult Sensory Profile*. San Antonio, TX: The Psychological Corporation.

Brown, C., Dunn, W., Tollefson, N., Cromwell, R. and Filion, D. (2001) 'The Adult Sensory Profile: Measuring patterns of sensory processing.' *American Journal of Occupational Therapy*, 55(1), 75–82.

Burns, A., Byrne, J., Ballard, C. and Holmes, C. (2002) 'Sensory stimulation in dementia: An effective option for managing behavioural problems.' *British Medical Journal*, 7(325), 1312–1313.

Collier, L. (2005) *The Sensory Assessment and Profiling Tool* [CD-ROM]. Manchester: Granada Learning.

Coq, J.-O. and Xerri, C. (2001) 'Sensorimotor experience modulates age-dependent alterations of the forepaw representation in the rat primary somatosensory cortex.' *Neuroscience*, 104(3), 705–715.

Corcoran, M. and Barrett, D. (1987) 'Using Sensory Integration Principles with Regressed Elderly Patients.' In Z. Mailloux (ed.) *Sensory Integrative Approaches in Occupational Therapy*. New York, NY: The Haworth Press.

Corso, J. (1971) 'Sensory processes and age effects in normal adults.' *Journal of Gerontology*, 26(1), 90–105.

Csikszentmihalyi, M. (1975) *Beyond Boredom and Anxiety: The Experience of Play in Work and Games*. San Francisco, CA: Jossey-Bass.

Csikszentmihalyi, M. and LeFevre, J. (1989) 'Optimal experience in work and leisure.' *Journal of Personality and Social Psychology*, 56(5), 815–822.

Dunn, W. (2001) 'The sensations of everyday life: Empirical, theoretical and pragmatic considerations.' *American Journal of Occupational Therapy*, 55(6), 608–620.

Dunn, W. and Brown, C. (1997) 'Factor analysis on the Sensory Profile from a national sample of children without disabilities.' *American Journal of Occupational Therapy*, 51(7), 490–495.

Dunn, W. and Westman, K. (1997) 'The Sensory Profile: The performance of a national sample of children without disabilities.' *American Journal of Occupational Therapy*, 51(1), 25–34.

Emerson, H. (1998) 'Flow and occupation: A review of the literature.' *Canadian Journal of Occupational Therapy*, 65(1), 37–44.

Hairston, W., Laurienti, P., Mishra, G., Burdette, J. and Wallace, M. (2003) 'Multisensory enhancement of localisation under conditions of induced myopia.' *Experimental Brain Research*, 152(3), 404–408.

Hall, G. and Buckwalter, K. (1987) 'Progressively lowered stress threshold: A conceptual model for care of adults with Alzheimer's disease.' *Archives of Psychiatric Nursing*, 1(6), 399–406.

Hebb, D. (1949) *The Organisation of Behaviour: A Neuropsychological Theory*. New York, NY: Wiley.

Heyn, P. (2003) 'The effect of a multisensory exercise program on engagement, behavior and selected physiological indexes in persons with dementia.' *American Journal of Alzheimer's Disease and Other Dementias*, 18(4), 247–251.

Jacobs, K. (1994) 'Flow and the occupational therapy practitioner.' *American Journal of Occupational Therapy*, 48(1), 989–996.

Keller, B., Morton, J., Thomas, V. and Potter, J. (1999) 'The effect of visual and hearing impairment on functional status.' *Journal of the American Geriatric Society*, 47, 1319–1325.

Kempermann, G., Gast, D. and Gage, F. (2002) 'Neuroplasticity in old age: Sustained fivefold induction of hippocampal neurogenesis by long-term environmental enrichment.' *Annals of Neurology*, 52(2), 135–143.

King, L. (1983) 'Sensory integration as neurophysiology.' *American Journal of Occupational Therapy*, 37(8), 568–569.

Kobayashi, S., Ohashi, Y. and Ando, S. (2002) 'Effects of enriched environments with different durations and starting times on learning capacity during aging in rats assessed by a refined procedure of the Hebb-Williams maze task.' *Journal of Neuroscience Research*, 70, 340–346.

Kovach, C. (2000) 'Sensoristasis and imbalance in persons with dementia.' *Journal of Nursing Scholarship*, 32(4), 379–384.

Kovach, C. and Magliocco, J. (1998) 'Late stage dementia and participation in therapeutic activities.' *Applied Nursing Research*, 11(4), 167–173.

Kovach, C. and Meyer Arnold, E. (1997) 'Preventing agitated behaviours during bath time.' *Geriatric Nursing*, 18(3), 112–114.

Laurienti, P., Burdette, J., Maljian, J. and Wallace, M. (2006) 'Enhanced multisensory integration in older adults.' *Neurobiology of Aging*, 27(8), 1155–1163.

Lawton, M. (1986) *Environment and Aging* (2nd edition). New York, NY: Albany.

Lomassese, S., Strambi, C., Strambi, A., Charpin, P. *et al.* (2000) 'Influence of environmental stimulation on neurogenesis in the adult insect brain.' *Journal of Neurobiology*, 45, 162–171.

Lu, L.-Q. and Zhao, C.-M. (2005) 'Enriched environment and neural plasticity.' *Chinese Journal of Clinical Rehabilitation*, 9(16), 141–143.

MacDonald, C. (2002) 'Back to the real sensory world our "care" has taken away.' *Journal of Dementia Care*, 10(1), 33–36.

McKhann, G. (2002) 'New neurons for aging brains.' *Annals of Neurology*, 52(2), 133–134.

Norberg, A., Melin, E. and Asplund, K. (1986) 'Reactions to music, touch and object presentation in the final stage of dementia: An exploratory study.' *International Journal of Nursing Studies*, 23, 315–323.

Perry, R. and Hodges, J. (1999) 'Attention and executive deficits in Alzheimer's disease: A critical review.' *Brain*, 122(3), 383–404.

Pohl, P., Dunn, W. and Brown, C. (2003) 'The role of sensory processing in the everyday lives of older adults.' *Occupational Therapy Journal of Research: Occupation, Participation and Health*, 23(3), 99–106.

Rochefort, C., Gheusi, G., Vincent, J. and Lledo, P. (2002) 'Enriched odour exposure increases the number of newborn neurons in the adult olfactory bulb and improves odour memory.' *Journal of Neuroscience*, 22(7), 2679–2689.

Roley, S., Clark, G., Bissell, J. and Brayman, S. (2003) 'Applying sensory integration framework in educationally related occupational therapy practice (2003 statement).' *American Journal of Occupational Therapy*, 57(6), 652–659.

Ross, M. and Burdick, D. (1981) *Sensory Integration*. Thorofare, NJ: Slack.

Sandeman, R. and Sandeman, D. (2000) 'Impoverished and enriched living conditions influence the proliferation and survival of neurons in crayfish brains.' *Journal of Neurobiology*, 45(4), 215–226.

Schaaf, R. and Miller, L. (2005) 'Occupational therapy using a sensory integrative approach for children with developmental disabilities.' *Mental Retardation Developmental Disabilities Research Reviews*, 11(2), 143–148.

Smith, S., Press, B., Koenig, K. and Kinnealey, M. (2005) 'Effects of sensory integration intervention on self-stimulating and self-injurious behaviors.' *American Journal of Occupational Therapy*, 59(4), 418–425.

Valentijn, S., van Boxtel, M., van Hooren, S., Bosma, H. *et al.* (2005) 'Change in sensory functioning predicts change in cognitive functioning: Results from a 6-year follow-up in the Maastricht Aging Study 168.' *Journal of the American Geriatrics Society*, 53(3), 374–380.

Voelkl, J. (1990) 'The challenge skill ratio of daily experiences among older adults residing in institutional environments.' *Therapeutic Recreation Journal*, 24(2), 7–17.

Voelkl, J., Ellis, G. and Walker, J. (2003) 'Go with the flow: How to help people have optimal recreation experiences.' *Parks and Recreation*, 38(8), 20–29.

Weale, R.A. (1963) 'New light on old eyes.' *Nature*, 198, 944–946.

Zegeer, L. (1986) 'The effects of sensory changes in older persons.' *Journal of Neuroscience Nursing*, 18(6), 325–332.

Zubek, J. (1969) *Sensory Deprivation: Fifteen Years of Research*. New York, NY: Appleton-Century-Crofts.

Chapter 11

SEEING RESULTS

AIMS AND RATIONALE OF THE QCS PAL INSTRUMENT

The reason for this guidebook is not simply to encourage readers to embark on a purely academic exercise to find out the level of a person's cognitive disability and the corresponding level of functional ability.

The recognition of the potential for cognitive rehabilitation for people with dementia in the NICE Guidelines for dementia (NG97) and in the World Health Organization 2030 Agenda for Sustainable Development enables care providers across health and social care to consider the inclusion of this approach in their services. In doing so, they need a baseline of the individual's cognitive and functional ability in order to plan the delivery as well as to monitor and review the impact of the rehabilitation approaches they are using. Because the QCS PAL Instrument is a standardized assessment, it can be the tool for identifying the baseline, using not only the overall level but also the raw data for each of the nine domains. The PAL Checklist can be repeated at intervals, for example before and after a programme of cognitive rehabilitation, in order to demonstrate the impact of the interventions on cognitive functional ability.

In addition, the PAL Engagement Measure provides a record of the person's engagement in a specific activity, supporting the planning and delivery of activity programmes as well as evidencing the impact of the service delivery to key stakeholders including regulators, commissioners, senior management teams and family members.

The guidebook is intended to enable caregivers and activity providers to enhance the experience of the person with cognitive impairment through an increased understanding of their abilities and the provision of appropriately presented occupations. When this occurs, there is often an effect on the person's psychological, social and cognitive experience. In other words, the person may not only have enhanced feelings of self-confidence and self-esteem, they may also experience a higher level of thinking and reasoning and of communication with others.

THE PERSON-CENTRED APPROACH

This is possible because of the close relationship between cognition, feeling and action. It is helpful to view these three states as the points of a triangle, each being separate from, but also interrelating with, the others. For example, low feelings cause every person to think, reason and act less efficiently; equally, negative thoughts cause low feelings and can stifle the ability to act effectively; and a lack of action can lead to low mood and negative thoughts. Knowledge of this triangle can be used by caregivers to raise the level of ability in all three areas by focusing on the two which are the most easily influenced in a person with cognitive impairment: feelings and actions.

This concept is at the heart of a person-centred approach to caring for people with dementia (Kitwood 1990) which is grounded in the theory that dementia is a disability caused not only by neurological impairment, but also by a damaging social psychology and undermining interactions with others, as well as a lack of opportunity for engagement in meaningful occupation.

Actions and activities can be used by caregivers as a vehicle for interaction. Communication which achieves close contact between the caregiver and the person with cognitive impairment will enhance the person's mood. In addition, if the activity or action is facilitated at the right level for the individual, feelings of self-confidence and self-esteem will also be experienced as the person is able to participate successfully. This type of success is not unusual and many caregivers report that the person they care for seems at times to improve beyond expectation.

RECORDING THE RESULTS OF ACTIVITIES

Giving real-life 'before and after' descriptions is an interesting way for caregivers to describe the results of their activity with an individual; but a story in itself may not be sufficient to convince others of the potential for improvement. Hard facts are sometimes needed. That is why it is helpful to keep records that show the progress of the person with cognitive impairment.

The PAL Engagement Measure has been validated as sensitive to change and shown to illustrate changes in engagement that are aligned with changes in behaviour, including relating to others, dexterity and emotional interaction. This new development of the QCS PAL Instrument battery of tools enables users to measure the outcome of specific activities in a reliable and structured way and also will alert the caregiver to the need to re-administer the PAL Checklist when significant improvements or deterioration in abilities is highlighted by the Engagement Measure. Information about an individual's cognitive status over time can also be gained from the raw data contained in the nine domains on the PAL Checklist. PAL users will need to decide the frequency of completing the PAL Checklist; this may be appropriate on a monthly or a quarterly basis but it should certainly be completed as part of any care or treatment plan review.

Caregivers of people with cognitive impairment in their own home may feel that record keeping is not for them, that it is only necessary for hospitals and care homes. But record keeping need not be complex or time consuming and it can have two major impacts on the experience of the people being cared for. First, if caregivers from all settings keep records, then they can contribute to research into effective ways of working with people with cognitive impairments. Second, if caregivers keep records and are actively seeking improvements in the experience of the person or people they care for, then they are maintaining an attitude of expectation, rather than one of acceptance that there is no scope for improvement. The negative culture of assuming an inevitable decline of the person with cognitive impairment, where the cause is viewed as progressive, such as in Alzheimer's disease, is now held to be harmful itself – it may become a self-fulfilling prophecy. If caregivers and the person being cared for accept this assumption, the person's psychological well-being is undermined, and this can adversely affect the person's physical health and functional ability. An expectation that positive caregiving can have a healing effect – where the person may improve to a higher level of cognition and ability – will change the whole culture of caring for this group of people.

REFERENCE

Kitwood, T. (1990) 'The dialectics of dementia: With particular reference to Alzheimer's disease.' *Ageing and Society*, 10(2), 177–196.

USING THE POOL ACTIVITY LEVEL (PAL) INSTRUMENT IN LEISURE ACTIVITIES

Sarah Mould and Jackie Pool

Chapter 12

INTRODUCTION TO PART 2

The engagement of people in meaningful activities provides the opportunity to be thinking, feeling and doing. It is this that is proven to be essential to physical and mental health. Activities that have meaning to the person, which excite their interest and also enable them to use a range of skills, optimize the potential for well-being.

Those who support people who have cognitive impairments caused by, for example, dementia, stroke or learning disability are all in a position to make it possible for the person for whom they care to engage in meaningful, enabling and fulfilling activity.

In order to understand the importance of the opportunity for activity, it is helpful to consider the model of 'emotional needs' described by Tom Kitwood (1997, pp.80–84). An understanding of the elements of this model often has an extremely profound impact on caregivers, not only in terms of what it is to be a human being, but what it must be like to live with a cognitive impairment.

The 'emotional needs' model describes six elements:

- Love (being the core)
- Attachment
- Comfort
- Identity
- Inclusion
- Occupation.

Caregivers realize the importance of all of these elements, including 'occupation', but somehow the words 'tasks', 'activities', 'achievement' and 'skills' can evolve into 'lack of time', 'too few staff', 'no resources', 'not part of my job', 'not valued', 'not trained'.

Caregivers need support from their team leaders and managers to become 'reflective practitioners' who consistently identify the following:

- We can enable a person to get dressed rather than 'get' a person dressed.
- Simply engaging in conversation with a person is undertaking an activity.
- Reading through a daily newspaper with the person being cared for is a valuable occupation.
- Playing a game of cards or facilitating some creative work with a person can be carried out without fear of chastisement because the laundry has not been put away.

Obstacles described by many caregivers are the lack of resources or equipment to carry out an activity and lack of guidance as to how to facilitate successful activities. Not all care services have access to occupational therapy services or the resources to employ activity coordinators.

Indeed, it may be reflected that this is part of the cause of the problem – do we need to rely on 'designated' people to undertake activities with service users?

The Pool Activity Level (PAL) Activity Profile will help caregivers and activity providers to understand the needs and skills of individuals in order to facilitate the right activity at the right time and at the right level. Once this is understood, perhaps caregivers will have the motivation and enthusiasm to facilitate meaningful engagement in personal care activity, domestic activity and leisure activity. Many caregivers have hobbies and interests that have helped them to develop a range of skills which they can bring to the workplace.

Activity providers can also utilize the PAL Activity Profile in order to facilitate engagement in programmed and spontaneous leisure activities that become meaningful as they are supported at the 'just right' level for the individual. The PAL Engagement Measure will support the activity provider to measure the impact of the activity they are facilitating on the individual and to monitor this over time, evidencing the well-being of the individual as well as the impact of their role.

People with cognitive impairments may have difficulty engaging in such activities, particularly if the activity is too demanding or not presented to the person in an understandable way. Care and activity staff trying to provide leisure activity programmes can be at a loss to know how to offer the activity to maximize success, or how to find equipment locally or nationally. The owners of the PAL Instrument, Quality Compliance Systems (QCS), have partnered with several activity resource companies to enable caregivers and activity providers to facilitate meaningful engagement in their activity resources by understanding how the PAL Instrument levels relate to their resources.

The National Activity Providers Association gives a wealth of advice and support, with ideas for activities. Relish Wellbeing has games and activities for people with dementia and an app for identifying the PAL level of individuals. The Daily Sparkle reminiscence newspaper and related activities also have a guide for enabling engagement in these at the assessed PAL level of ability of the individual.

In addition, Part 2 of this QCS PAL book guides caregivers and activity providers to improve their skills when facilitating leisure activities. Ideas for four activity packs are set out in the next four chapters. A selection of possible activities to be included is listed for each pack. This is not an exhaustive list and caregivers may choose to omit some and to add others. Possible sources for each activity are identified, but caregivers may choose to search other means of obtaining them.

Each chapter includes guidance on carrying out a range of activities with individuals who have different levels of ability as revealed by the completion of the PAL Instrument Checklist. The four activity packs are:

- table-top games
- social games
- creative activities
- sensory activities.

REFERENCES

Kitwood, T. (1997) *Dementia Reconsidered: The Person Comes First*. Buckingham: Open University Press.
Daily Sparkle reminiscence newspaper: www.dailysparkle.co.uk
National Activity Providers Association: https://napa-activities.co.uk
Relish Wellbeing: www.relish-life.com

Chapter 13

TABLE-TOP GAMES ACTIVITY PACK

SUGGESTED CONTENTS

- Large-print Scrabble game
- Large-piece jigsaw (x 2)
- Large-print playing cards
- Large-size playing cards
- Card holder (for four)
- The board game 'Frustration'
- Large-piece dominoes

POSSIBLE SOURCES

NRS Healthcare: www.nrshealthcare.co.uk/health-aids-personal-care/games-craft

The Consortium: www.consortiumeducation.com/care/activities/dementia-activities

Winslow Resources: www.winslowresources.com/rehabilitation-and-functioning/dementia-meaningful-activities.html

INTRODUCTION

This pack will be appropriate for those who have been established as having ability at either the *planned* or *exploratory* activity level using the QCS Pool Activity Level (PAL) Instrument.

The activities within this pack can be used with a single person or a small group. The number of people involved in each activity will be determined by the type of activity, skills and abilities of the participants, the environment/room available and the availability of care staff to facilitate.

Guidance regarding the number of people who can engage with each activity is given within this chapter.

The length of time the activity lasts will be determined by the response of the individuals and will rely on the facilitator's observational skills to determine when the activity should cease.

People with moderate to severe cognitive impairments may have a very short attention span and the activity may only be appropriate for a few minutes. One of the benefits of some of the activities in this pack is that they do not need to be put away when someone has finished using them. Where possible, the activity can be left out so that the person can return to it when they feel like engaging with it again. This opportunity for spontaneity is extremely valuable when working with people with cognitive impairments.

UNDERSTANDING THE ABILITY OF THE PERSON

Understanding what the person can and cannot do is vital to the success of the activity. If the activity is too difficult, a person may become anxious or frustrated. If the activity is too easy, they may feel unmotivated to take part.

The activities within this pack are likely to be very familiar to people. However, it is essential that care staff understand at which level the individual is functioning in order that the right amount of support and facilitation is offered and the activity is presented in the right way.

The activities require a range of cognitive skills: attention and concentration, problem solving, memory, planning, as well as awareness of rules, visual and symbolic recognition, numerical and word-finding skills and fine motor dexterity. The way that people with cognitive impairments are supported to undertake and enjoy these activities hinges on the skill, understanding and knowledge of the care staff.

Never allow yourself to find that you are playing *for* the person rather than *with* them.

Planned activity level

At a *planned* activity level the person can work towards completing a task, but may not be able to solve any problems that arise while in the process. They will be able to look in obvious places for objects needed but may not be able to search beyond the usual places. A caregiver assisting someone at this level will need to keep their sentences short and avoid using words like objects needed, which tend to be used to link two sentences together into a more complex one. Caregivers will also need to stand by to help solve any problems should they arise. People functioning at a planned activity level are able to carry out tasks which achieve a tangible result.

Exploratory activity level

At an *exploratory* activity level the person can carry out very familiar tasks in familiar surroundings. However, at this level people are more concerned with the effect of doing the activity rather than the consequence, and may not have an end result in mind. Therefore, a creative and spontaneous approach by caregivers to tasks is helpful. If an activity involves more than two or three tasks, a person at this level will need help in breaking the activity into manageable chunks. Directions need to be kept very simple and the use of memory aids such as task lists, calendars and labelling of frequently used items can be very helpful.

LARGE-PRINT SCRABBLE GAME

Scrabble is a word game for two, three or four players. Play consists of forming interlocking words, crossword fashion, on the 'Scrabble' playing board, using letter tiles with various score values. The objective of the game is to get the highest score.

Each player competes by using their tile combinations and locations that take best advantage of letter values and premium squares on the board. There is a very thorough instructions booklet with the game which care staff are advised to read and have to hand when playing.

In this large-print edition, the letters on the tiles are enlarged to enable players with cognitive impairments to have the maximum opportunity for visual recognition and thence letter identification.

Of course, players may also have a visual impairment, so the enlarged letters will be equally valuable.

You will know which of the people you provide care for are likely to enjoy Scrabble. Consider the person's:

- personality – do they enjoy word games or crosswords?
- biography – has the person always been interested in language and vocabulary? Are they a past 'Scrabble champion'? Did they play the game with their friends and family?
- cognitive ability – what is the person's attention span? Do they recognize words and letters, do they have a vocabulary of words within their memory? Could they solve problems?
- social factors – do they enjoy company? Are there people to whom they seem to relate well and who have similar interests? Are they aware of social rules such as turn taking? Are they easily distracted?
- physical factors – does the person have the fine motor skills necessary to manipulate the letter tiles?

These and many more facets of the person need to be considered when inviting them to play Scrabble so that it is made as rewarding and enjoyable an experience as possible.

When playing with a person at the *planned* activity level, be conscious of how you present the game. Ask if they have played it or seen it before. People at this activity level may have difficulty in grasping the instructions if they are described in full. Break the instructions down; for example, the booklet with the game which care staff can advise on: 'I'll put the tiles in this bag. Please take seven [count them out with the person]. Put them on this rack', and so on.

Constantly gauge the person's response to the activity and level of instruction and adapt your approach as required.

People at the *planned* activity level will have difficulty in solving problems as they arise. Ask the person if they will allow you to help them and suggest to them what they might do. Leave the decision up to the person – it may not have been the decision you would make. (Remember: you are playing with them, not for them.)

Sometimes people with cognitive impairments may have word-finding difficulties and may create words. Be advised by the game rules and the other players as to whether a word is acceptable or not. Although some debate is healthy, argument is not to be encouraged and you may need to mediate.

People who are at the *planned* activity level will be looking for an outcome; an end product to the activity in terms of a winner. Gauge how long to play the game in order that the participants have an opportunity to identify a winner, end the game and be congratulated on their performance.

When playing with someone at the *exploratory* activity level, be mindful that the end result will not be as important to them. They may enjoy examining the tiles and the textures of the game components. Instructions, again, must be very simple and will require repetition.

You may consider working as a team with a member of care staff to provide support to the person at this level and to help maintain the focus required.

Be prepared for and welcome spontaneity. Certain words may elicit reminiscence or recitation of a song or poetry – welcome this.

As facilitators, you must use all your skills to observe the response of the participants, adapt your approach if required, offer help if requested and maintain the momentum of the activity, but at the participants' pace. It may be helpful to set a time to play to and identify the winner at that point. However, people at an *exploratory* activity level of ability may not be so concerned with the end result of winning as the enjoyment of taking part.

On completion of the game, thank everyone for joining in. They may want to assist you to put the Scrabble away. (As there are many small components to the game, it is not advisable to leave it out.)

LARGE-PIECE JIGSAW

Working on a jigsaw puzzle has long been associated with peaceful contemplation and relaxation. (There may be occasional outbursts of frustration too!) Some may consider jigsaw puzzles a childlike pursuit, but look in any hobby store and you will find countless jigsaws surrounded by adults who enjoy the fascination of completion and the vibrancy of the picture.

Completing a jigsaw can be a solitary pursuit if that is someone's preference, or can be an opportunity for a pair to engage in true teamwork as one mind.

The jigsaw puzzles suggested for this activity pack are composed of large pieces but have pictures that are appropriate for adults. They are designed to enable people to achieve success through maximizing opportunities for visual recognition, problem solving and manipulation, among other cognitive skills. The large pieces are also helpful if people have difficulty with fine motor skills.

Again, your knowledge of the person will indicate whether a jigsaw puzzle would be a suitable activity. However, if someone shows an interest but has never done a jigsaw before, do not preclude them from taking part – they may have discovered a new pastime.

Ascertain that the person would like to attempt a jigsaw. Consider the person's:

- personality – do they enjoy puzzles?
- biography – has the person always been interested in table-top games?
- cognitive ability – what is the person's attention span, do they recognize colour and shapes, can they solve problems?
- social factors – do they enjoy company, are there people to whom the person seems to relate well and who have similar interests? Is the person aware of social rules such as turn taking, or would they prefer to complete a jigsaw alone? Are they easily distracted?
- physical factors – does the person have the fine motor skills necessary to manipulate the pieces?

If the person is at the *planned* activity level, they may prefer to be left alone to complete the jigsaw independently. (Make sure they do not find it so easy as to feel patronized.)

If the person is at the *exploratory* activity level, ask if they would permit you to help them.

Clearly, if the person would prefer to do it themselves, encourage this. In both cases, maintain a position where you will be available for help if needed.

You may like to set the jigsaw up so that it can be left out after the person has finished with it, either completed or uncompleted. This will maximize the opportunity for spontaneity, the person can place a piece almost as they walk by, or become engaged with it for a longer period.

You may wish to consider purchasing a variety of jigsaw puzzles to suit the different needs and abilities of the people for whom you care. It would be useful to have a range of pictures that relate to individuals' interests.

PLAYING CARDS AND CARD HOLDERS

Card games are very familiar to a wide range of people and have been a source of enjoyment for centuries. The appearance of a pack of cards – the colours, suits, design and shape – is recognized by people throughout the world. People with cognitive impairment are likely to recognize a pack of cards by using their visual recognition skills and memory; possibly they have been a lifelong card player, either as a solitary pursuit or in a team, at a bridge club or the casino, or perhaps a game of cards was a regular activity within the home or in the pub.

Two sets of playing cards are suggested within this pack: a regular-size pack of cards with large print and a large-size pack of cards. Your knowledge of the person will determine which of the packs you use and how you use it.

When engaging a person in a game of cards you need to consider the person's:

- personality – is this something in which they show an interest? Have they initiated the idea of playing cards? (You may wish to consider having the packs of cards in view, perhaps on a table or cupboard, to enable individuals to find them and perhaps instigate a game.)
- biography – do they have prior experience of playing cards?
- cognitive ability – is the person able to engage in a game independently, or will they require assistance to maintain the rules of play and to problem solve?
- social factors – do they enjoy company? Are there people to whom they seem to relate well and who have similar interests? Are they aware of social rules such as turn taking? Would they prefer games for one person, such as patience? Are they easily distracted?
- physical factors – does the person have the fine motor skills necessary to manipulate the cards and the larger movement ability to reach across a card table?

People at the *planned* activity level are likely to be able to engage in a game independently if the game is familiar to them and they have a good attention span. You may consider the following card games:

- Pontoon or 21
- Black Jack
- Rummy
- Canasta
- Poker
- Patience
- Bridge.

If a person with cognitive impairment could teach the game to a caregiver this would be a highly motivating and enriching experience for the person. You may wish to consider if a caregiver needs to be involved. Perhaps a person could be set up with a game of Patience to engage with on their own. If it is possible to leave the card game out, the person can leave and come back to it if they choose.

A caregiver need not be involved at all. If you are in a residential care home or day service, you could introduce residents or service users to each other in order that they could share their enthusiasm for card games. There should be a quiet area where a game of cards can be played. Consider the environment carefully to minimize distractions associated with noise, poor lighting and interruptions.

The regular pack of cards has large print which will maximize the opportunity for a person with visual impairment or difficulty with visual recognition to participate in a game.

Card holders are also recommended for this pack because they are of benefit to people who have difficulty holding a hand of cards. You can also place the hand of cards in a card holder to enable the person to see each card more easily. The large pack of cards enhances this even further, though you may wish to use this pack in a different way. People at the *exploratory* activity level may enjoy a team game based on the old television programme 'Play Your Cards Right'.

'Play Your Cards Right'

1. You will need a method whereby you can place the large playing cards upright. (If you have a flipchart you can place the cards in the groove at the bottom so that they lean against the board. If you have a fairly narrow piece of furniture, you could place the cards on this so that they lean against the wall. Otherwise you could place the cards flat on a table but make sure everyone can see them.)
2. Shuffle the cards and place six of them face down so that the back of the cards is showing.
3. Identify a quiz master and two teams.
4. Ask each team in turn a quiz question.
5. If they get the question right they can move on to the six cards prepared.
6. Turn the first card over. Advise the team that they need to decide whether the next card will be higher or lower than this card.
7. If the team correctly predicts whether the card will be higher or lower, allocate ten points and move on to the next card.
8. If the team correctly predicts all six cards, allocate them an extra 100 points.
9. Clear this row of cards and replace with six new ones, placed face down.
10. Move on to the next team and repeat the process.
11. The winning team is the one with the highest score after all the playing cards have been used.

Game rules

- If the first card turned over is the same as the first card in the line, the team can choose to change it.
- If, further down the line, the card is the same as the previous one, the team has lost as it is neither higher nor lower than the previous card. (You may wish to use the catchphrase 'You get nothing for a pair...not in this game!' as Bruce Forsyth did in the game show.)
- If the team incorrectly predicts the turn of the card, the other team can take over and try to complete the line. If they make an error, pass the turn back to the other team.
- Do not use the jokers. Aces are high (higher than the king).

Try to get into the spirit of the game (this will be very easy), with lots of 'oohs' and 'aahs' at the turn of the cards to increase the anticipation and tension.

Other card games

You could use the large cards to play Patience, but you will need a very large table! If you would like to invest in a second pack of large playing cards you could use this to play Pairs. Sort the cards from both packs into pairs. Lay these randomly on a table face down, no more than eight pairs. The person with cognitive impairment is asked to turn a card over and identify it. Then ask the person to turn over a second card. If the cards match, remove both from the table. If they do not match, turn both over, face down, and continue. The game is over when all cards are paired.

Or you could play the perennial favourite Snap. Each player has a pack of cards and places them on the table in front of them face down. In turn, each player places a card face up on the table. If the cards match, the first person to shout 'Snap' wins the whole stack of cards. The winner is the person who ends up with all the cards.

The response of the individuals playing will determine how long the game of cards will last. Remember that people with cognitive impairment may have a short attention span, so one game may be enough.

Do not correct the actions the person takes if the person chooses to do something that you may not have done. Use tact, verbal suggestion and shared problem solving to support someone who is making errors which appear to be affecting their sense of well-being and enjoyment.

Monitor for signs of confusion, lack of interest or distraction and adapt your approach accordingly. The objective of the game is enjoyment and a sense of achievement. Again, do not patronize the person by taking over or playing for them, and make sure that the level is correct for each individual so that they do not find the game too hard or too easy.

Thank the participants for joining in the game and allow some time for reflection.

You may like to consider setting up a 'cards club' as a regular weekly event, if appropriate.

THE BOARD GAME 'FRUSTRATION'

Board games are a popular pastime in homes and clubs throughout the world. Competition, problem solving and fun are all key components in participating in a board game.

The game Frustration which is suggested in this pack makes use of several cognitive functions and is therefore suited to people at the *planned* and *exploratory* activity levels. Because the dice is enclosed within the board, it is also less likely to be lost.

The amount of support and guidance required will vary according to the activity level of the person and their skills and interests. It is important, in a pastime such as this, that you do not mix participants from different activity levels. At a *planned* activity level, the participants are likely to require ongoing reminding of the rules of play and guidance perhaps as to what to do for each move, as they are likely to have difficulty with problem solving. Participants at this level may be quite competitive, therefore it is important that they do not feel 'held back' by someone who is at a different activity level and who may not be able to respond as quickly or who does not maintain interest throughout.

At an *exploratory* activity level, the participants are likely to be less concerned with the outcome of the game and more interested in taking part and the process. Again, it is likely that the participants will require verbal and gestural prompting to maintain their focus on the game and to be able to sequence each step effectively. It is therefore important that they are not playing with someone at a different activity level as they may be responded to in a negative way if they do not maintain the pace of the game, or make 'mistakes'.

The game has detailed instructions of play on the back of the box. Take time to read through them and understand them, so that as a facilitator you can maintain the focus and momentum of the activity (have the instructions next to you just in case!). Consider the person's:

- personality – is this something that the person shows an interest in?

- biography – do they have prior experience of playing this game or other similar games such as Ludo?
- cognitive ability – is the person able to engage in a game independently or will they require assistance to maintain the rules of play and to problem solve? Can the person recognize colour? They will need to do so in order to distinguish between the four colours used in the game.
- social factors – do they enjoy company? Are there people to whom they seem to relate well and who have similar interests? Are they aware of social rules such as turn taking? Are they easily distracted?
- physical factors – does the person have the movement skills and strength to push the dice shaker and the larger movement ability to reach across the board? (It may be appropriate to consider teams of pairs – one participant and one caregiver per team to support each other in cognitive and physical process needs.)

On completion of the game, thank everyone for joining in and allow time for reflection. The participants may wish to help you put the game away.

LARGE-PIECE DOMINOES

The large-piece dominoes included in this pack are suited to the needs of people with cognitive and sensory impairment. The size of the dominoes ensures that maximum opportunity is provided for people with visual, numerical and symbolic recognition difficulties to participate in this pastime. The dominoes are suitable for people with visual impairment, the black dots on the pale background making identification quite easy. People with manual dexterity problems will also find the large-size dominoes easier to manipulate.

The instructions for play are usually included in the dominoes box and are easy to follow.

You will have a good understanding of the skills and interests of the person with cognitive impairment in order to know whether they will enjoy a game of dominoes and at what level to present the activity.

A game of dominoes is an excellent activity for promoting social interaction too, providing an opportunity for engagement between players. They may have reminiscences of playing dominoes before or may like to share stories of pastimes they have enjoyed. Encourage this.

At the *planned* activity level, it is likely that the person will be able to participate in the activity independently by playing with one other person or a group of people. The person may require occasional prompting with the placing of the dominoes. Offer assistance when requested, and do not be intrusive; for example, if someone is having difficulty locating or choosing a domino, ask if they will allow you to look at their dominoes and facilitate their decision-making process in choosing a domino. Let the person place the domino on the table – do not do this for them unless they ask you to. Offer positive reinforcement throughout the activity.

At the *exploratory* activity level, the person may need more support and facilitation with identification of the domino and knowing where to place it on the table. Again, do not be intrusive. You may like to consider playing the game in pairs to enhance focus and enjoyment based on feelings of agency and success. Let the response of the participants guide you as to how long to play. The whole experience should be relaxing and enjoyable for all, so make sure that you play in an environment as free from distraction as possible.

Thank the players for participating in the activity and allow some time for reflection.

Chapter 14

SOCIAL GAMES ACTIVITY PACK

SUGGESTED CONTENTS

- Parachute
- Ring-toss set
- Sing-along playlist, audio streaming or karaoke machine and song book/sheets
- Skittles set
- Bean-bag target

POSSIBLE SOURCES

AlzProducts: www.alzproducts.co.uk

NRS Healthcare: www.nrshealthcare.co.uk/health-aids-personal-care/games-craft

The Consortium: www.consortiumeducation.com/care/activities/dementia-activities

Winslow Resources: www.winslowresources.com/rehabilitation-and-functioning/dementia-meaningful-activities.html

INTRODUCTION

This pack will be appropriate for those who have been established as having ability at either the *planned*, *exploratory* or *sensory* activity level using the QCS Pool Activity Level (PAL) Instrument.

As the title of this pack would suggest, the activities contained within it are intended to be used with a group of people. The number of people within the group will be determined by the type of activity, the skills and abilities of the participants, the environment/room available and the availability of care staff to facilitate.

Guidance as to numbers for each activity is given within this chapter. The length of time the activity lasts will be determined by the response of the individuals and will rely on the facilitator's observational skills to determine when the activity should cease. Though these are group activities, it is essential that each individual's response is monitored to observe signs of well- or ill-being.

Some of these activities are quite physical, so facilitators need to be aware of the individual's stamina, mobility and physical health needs. Be aware, too, that people with moderate to severe cognitive impairment may have a very short attention span.

UNDERSTANDING THE ABILITY OF THE PERSON

Understanding what the person can and cannot do is vital to the success of the activity. If the activity is too difficult, a person may become anxious or frustrated. If the activity is too easy, the person may feel unmotivated to take part. The nature of these activities also requires that people engage with others socially. People do not respond well when they feel pressured to take part in an activity when they do not wish to. Some people may feel uncomfortable or embarrassed in front of other people. Some may not be used to the company of others. Of course, some people thrive on social contact and all the positive reinforcement this can bring. People with moderate to severe cognitive impairment may not be aware of 'social norms' and rules. This will therefore require facilitators to observe the group dynamics and adjust the activity if required to ensure that the aims of the activities are achieved.

Planned activity level

At a *planned* activity level the person can work towards completing a task but may not be able to solve any problems that arise while in the process. They will be able to look in obvious places for objects needed, but may not be able to search beyond the usual places. Caregivers assisting someone at this level will need to keep their sentences short and avoid using words like 'and' or 'but' which tend to be used to link two sentences together into a more complex one. Caregivers will also need to stand by to help solve any problems should they arise. People functioning at a planned activity level are able to carry out tasks that achieve a tangible result.

Exploratory activity level

At an *exploratory* activity level the person can carry out very familiar tasks in familiar surroundings. However, at this level people are more concerned with the effect of doing the activity than in the consequence and may not have an end result in mind. Therefore, a creative and spontaneous approach by caregivers to tasks is helpful. If an activity involves more than two or three tasks, a person at this level will need help in breaking the activity into manageable chunks. Directions need to be made very simple and the use of memory aids such as task lists, calendars and labelling of frequently used items can be very helpful.

Sensory activity level

At a *sensory* activity level the person may not have many thoughts or ideas about carrying out an activity: they are mainly concerned with the sensation and with moving their body in response to those sensations. People at this level can be guided to carry out single-step tasks such as sweeping or winding wool. More complex activities can only be carried out when directed one step at a time. Therefore, caregivers need to ensure that the person at this activity level has the opportunity to experience a wide variety of sensations and to carry out one-step tasks. Directions to maximize this opportunity need to be kept very simple and be reinforced by demonstrating the action required.

PARACHUTE

The word 'exercise' often conjures up images of going to the gym or jogging – not always possible, appropriate or desired. However, participation in physical exercise is essential to maintain health and well-being. Evidence shows that participation in exercise has psychological benefits too. It can also be fun!

A parachute as a means of exercise and social engagement may not have been your first consideration, but for people at both *exploratory* and *sensory* activity levels, this entirely suits their needs for enjoyment of the process of an activity that has simple, straightforward steps and sensory input.

Why a parachute?

- Parachute activity promotes cooperation. Everyone shares the same objects at the same time, so working together rather than against each other is the aim.
- The parachute naturally forms a circle, so everyone will form around this and be able to see each other, enhancing awareness of others.
- There are no losers in parachute games.
- Parachute games are flexible in terms of the amount of time used and opportunities for spontaneity.
- The parachute is lightweight, and once unfurled is ready to use.
- Parachutes lend themselves to the imagination. This may be the first time that someone has even seen a parachute, let alone worked with one. This rare sight can therefore trigger the creative senses.
- The facilitator/s actively participate too.

One is never too old to play, but consideration must be given to older people with cognitive impairment who may require this activity to be presented in a different way.

Consider the person's:

- personality – do they enjoy social gatherings and physical activity?
- biography – have they handled a parachute before? (Be prepared for some reminiscence about this before the activity begins.)
- cognitive ability – is the person able to maintain attention and sustain their hold of the parachute?
- social factors – do they enjoy company? Are there people to whom they seem to relate well?
- physical factors – is the person in a wheelchair? Do they have respiratory or cardiac problems? Do they have arthritis or any inflammatory disease? Do they have tender skin? Do they have osteoporosis or have they recently suffered a bone injury? Do they have difficulty with balance and coordination as a result of a stroke or neurological impairment?

It may not be possible to undertake parachute games outdoors, therefore consideration of the environment is essential. There should be space for six to eight people to form a circle in the room. The ceiling height should be sufficient for the parachute activities, and the needs of people who use wheelchairs should be considered.

Suggested session plan

You may wish to spend some time exploring the parachute with the group before you begin the games.

1. Explain to the group that you have a parachute. Remove it from the bag and allow it

to spread out over the floor. It may be appropriate for all the group participants to be seated in stable, straight-backed chairs.

2. Enable each of the participants to feel the texture of the parachute by placing some of the material on their lap and encouraging them to touch and hold it. Monitor each person's response. If the person shows signs of distress or lack of interest or requests not to join in, allow them to leave the group and enable them to choose whether they would like to sit and watch or do something else individually.

3. Support each individual to hold one or two of the handles. Consider the number of facilitators required and where they are placed in terms of providing the optimum amount of support to individuals.

4. Begin by encouraging the participants to slowly lift their arms up and down until the parachute is inflating and deflating rhythmically.

5. Play some appropriate music in the background to encourage pace and to set the mood. Constantly monitor the response of the individuals. There can be quite a draught when the parachute deflates. Also be aware of any expressions of pain or stiffness.

6. Allow the group to rest the parachute on their laps, still holding on to it.

7. Facilitate the group to pass the parachute round – still keeping it spread out, encouraging hold and release of the parachute handles. Pass it back the other way. Check for responses – hopefully there will be laughter and verbal and non-verbal communication. Mirror these responses.

8. Facilitate the group to raise and lower their arms alternately as quickly as they are able, to give a ripple effect to the parachute.

9. Follow this again with gentle raising and lowering of arms, as in step 4.

10. Allow the group to rest for a few moments. Ask how they are feeling and check that they are happy to continue.

11. Facilitate the group to lift and lower their arms again. Inform them that you are going to throw a very light ball onto the parachute and that their task is not to let it fall off. As the parachute inflates, throw a light, brightly coloured ball onto the parachute. (It is helpful if it's of a contrasting colour.) Encourage the group to use their hand-eye coordination to lift their bit of the parachute to keep the ball on it. Check for responses and over-exuberance, which can be quite frightening and off-putting for some people.

If the group is happy to continue you might like to try one of the games described below. The more familiar you become with the games, the more likely that you will be able to adapt this plan according to the needs and preferences of your group members.

Mushroom

Everyone holds the parachute taut. On the count of three, everyone lifts the parachute high above their heads. A giant mushroom is formed. Encourage the participants to watch as the parachute slowly descends.

(If you have enough space or are using the parachute outside you could play the 'Floating Mushroom' by asking the group to let go of the parachute when it is fully lifted above their heads.)

Igloo

This is a game for people standing or in wheelchairs. On the count of three, everyone lifts the parachute high above their heads like a mushroom. Ask them to take a couple of steps in – or assist the person in the wheelchair by pushing them forward – and to bring the parachute down behind them with everyone facing each other inside.

Parachute golf

Invite the participants to hold the parachute fairly taut. Throw a ball or several balls into the parachute with the instruction that the participants work together to get the balls to go through the hole in the middle of the parachute. (Ensure that the balls are smaller than the hole in the parachute!)

Make sure that you end the group activity by approaching each individual in turn and thanking them for joining in. Take the parachute from them and begin to roll the parachute up in readiness for putting it away. Spend a few moments of quiet reflection together or play some relaxing music to enable the participants to feel calm and relaxed and to return heart rates to normal!

RING-TOSS SET

Many people are familiar with the game Hoopla. This next activity may therefore have some familiar associations for the participants.

If necessary, prepare the target before you invite people to join in a game.

This activity can be played with any number of people, but it is recommended that there are no more than six to eight in the group. It becomes increasingly difficult for people with cognitive impairment to maintain focus and interest in an activity if they are not engaged for most of the time. Waiting for other people to take their turn in an activity can be frustrating and boring for some, who may leave the activity either cognitively or physically.

Consider the person's:

- personality – do they enjoy social gatherings and physical activity?
- biography – have they played similar games before? (Some people may relate this to childhood and may not wish to play a 'childish' game – this should be respected.)
- cognitive ability – is the person able to maintain attention and sustain their participation in the competition?
- social factors – do they enjoy company? Are there people to whom the person seems to relate well?
- physical factors – is the person in a wheelchair? Do they have respiratory or cardiac problems? Do they have arthritis or any inflammatory disease? Do they have osteoporosis or have they recently suffered a bone injury? Do they have difficulty with balance and coordination as a result of a stroke or neurological impairment? You will need to ensure that the participants have fairly good manual dexterity, balance and visual skills. It may be more beneficial for the participants to play this game sitting down.

Arrange the group in a circle of comfortable chairs and place the target in the middle of the floor within the circle. Use your judgement and knowledge of the participants to gauge how far the target needs to be from them.

This is a competitive game, but be mindful of facilitating each individual within the group to experience success, no matter what their ability. You can facilitate the game as a group of individuals, but it is much more fun, and more sociable, to facilitate the group in teams. You can ask each team to give themselves a name which will emphasize identity and place participants in a mutually cooperative situation of support.

Demonstrate how the game is played and agree any rules with the participants, such as the number of rounds, whether the target can be moved, when to have a break or refreshments.

You will need a score board.

Toss a coin to decide which team will begin. Begin round 1.

The first player in the team is handed the rings and facilitated to throw them towards the target, aiming to achieve a high score by getting the rings over the dowels. At the *planned* activity level you may need to verbally encourage the person to do this; at an *exploratory* activity level you may need to physically demonstrate a throwing action; and at a *sensory* activity level you may need to guide the person to make a throwing action by placing your hand over theirs. Record the first player's score and move on to the first player in the next team. Ensure that each player in each team has a go and record the combined total of all the players as the team scores. Move on to round 2.

At the end of the game, total the scores for each round and announce the winning team.

Ensure that throughout the game you are offering lots of encouragement through verbal and non-verbal reinforcement for each individual as they take their turn.

Remember that for people at the *planned* activity level it is possible that they will be quite competitive among themselves as individuals and within their teams. This will help to maintain focus for the participants, but they may require assistance to problem solve if anything 'unplanned' happens. At the *exploratory* activity level, the action of throwing the rings and involvement in the social camaraderie of the activity is likely to be more fulfilling than the end result of the game. For those at the *sensory* activity level, the sensation of the rings in their hands, the action of throwing and the audible enjoyment of the activity will be stimulating.

Thank the group for their participation. Put the ring-toss equipment to one side.

You may wish to end the session with some relaxing music, allowing the participants to chat quietly and reflect on the session.

SING-ALONG

Singing is an invigorating activity which usually promotes a happy feeling, provides a means of releasing tensions and is often evocative of past experiences and emotions (Mercer 2006).

As part of everyday life, music is more than just a noise, and often holds personal significance. Music for Dementia is a national campaign to make music an integral part of dementia care in the UK, recognizing the power of music for people at all levels, and its m4d Radio is a group of five themed radio stations available 24 hours a day, 365 days a year playing music that evokes memories. Sing-along activities can be presented to people at the *planned* and *exploratory* activity levels and simple enjoyment and movement to the music can be enjoyed by people at any of the four PAL levels of ability.

When organizing a sing-along, consider the person's:

- personality – what type of music do they enjoy? Music is a very personal choice. One person's delight may be another's racket, so selecting the 'right' songs while catering for a range of tastes is important.

- biography – it is likely that some of the songs may provoke recall and reminiscence of earlier days and experiences. This is extremely useful in terms of engagement and communication. Be mindful of strong emotion, which may be expressed in tears – of joy or sorrow. Be prepared to support individuals in the expression of these emotions, being aware that they are among others.
- cognitive ability – does the person have difficulty with speech? It is often found that people with profound verbal language impairment may still be able to sing fluently. Can the person recognize the words on the song sheet? If the song is familiar this may not matter as the words may come back to them when they hear the music.
- social factors – is the person comfortable singing in a group, do they prefer just to listen or are they a 'performer'?
- physical factors – does the person have a hearing impairment? Do they need to wear a hearing aid? Do they need to be positioned closely to the speaker or beside someone with a strong singing voice to enable them to hear? Does the person have a visual impairment? Many song books are in large print, but may need to be made larger for some participants.

When organizing a sing-along, explain to the individuals what is going to happen and verify that they are happy to participate. Seat the group in comfortable chairs, preferably in a circle so that everyone can see each other and feel included.

You will have decided which songs you are going to use and have set the music up so that it will begin at the correct place.

If you decide to make photocopies of the book or song sheets, please refer to the copyright regulations at the front of the song book regarding reproduction. (Your organization can contact the Copyright Licensing Agency Ltd on 020 7400 3100 for advice about fees.)

Tell the group the name of the first song which they will be singing. Ensure that everyone is prepared and start the music.

The facilitator/s have a key role in encouraging the group to sing and should always feel comfortable to start the singing and ensure that the group members are singing too, by using facial expression and hand gestures such as conducting.

Sing the first song, all the while monitoring the response of the participants to ensure that they feel comfortable. Participants must not be forced to join in; listening is an equally important activity. At the end of the song, pause the music and ask the group if they enjoyed it. If the group is happy to continue, play the next song. Gauge continuously the response of the participants. Some may spontaneously stand and dance – encourage this if it is safe to do so.

When all the songs have been sung, the participants might like to choose a song to sing again. Again, be mindful of the responses of the group. If a participant appears distressed, offer reassurance but do not assume that they want to leave the group – check with them.

Thank everyone for joining in. Consider suggesting a regular sing-along and agree when to meet again. Play some gentle music to enable the participants to relax, or by gauging the response of the group play the music again, allowing the participants to join in spontaneously.

People at a sensory activity level may like to listen to the songs. It is unlikely that they will follow the words from the book, but they may sing spontaneously, or hum. They may also enjoy using some musical instruments such as tambourines or maracas to play along to the music.

SKITTLES SET

As a social pastime, many people participate in bowling, either at a skittles alley or on the bowling green. Bowling is an enjoyable activity and, by its very nature, a social one.

A bowling set can be utilized by people who are functioning at the planned, exploratory or sensory activity levels.

The number of people you engage in this activity will be determined by their interests, preferences and physical abilities. You will also need a lot of space and a smooth floor of wood, lino or close-weave carpet.

Consider the person's:

- personality – do they enjoy social gatherings and physical activity?
- biography – have they played bowls before, perhaps they have belonged to a club?
- cognitive ability – is the person able to maintain attention on the game and to follow the rules? Can they let go of the bowling ball to roll it towards the skittles or the jack?
- social factors – do they enjoy company? Are there people to whom they seem to relate well?
- physical factors – is the person in a wheelchair? Do they have respiratory or cardiac problems? Do they have arthritis or any inflammatory disease? Do they have osteo-porosis or have they recently suffered a bone injury? Do they have difficulty with balance and coordination as a result of a stroke or neurological impairment?

In order to set up the activity, ensure that the area is hazard free and that you have lots of room for people to move around.

Set up the skittles in a triangular formation, one skittle at the front, then two placed behind adjacent to each other, then three in a line at the back. Decide how far the distance between the bowler and the skittles will be and place a marker of some kind to indicate where the bowler will stand. This will form your 'bowling alley'.

Place a row of chairs either side of the alley facing each other. This will be where your teams will sit. The distance between the chairs will be determined by the physical needs of the participants.

You will need a scoreboard to record each individual's score and thence the team score which will be totalled at the end. There may be a person who does not want to be involved in the bowling, but who would enjoy being the score master.

Introduce the activity to the participants and demonstrate what they need to do (to bowl each of the balls in turn in an attempt to knock down as many skittles as possible).

Facilitate the participants to form teams and encourage them to name their team. Toss a coin to identify which team will start. Encourage the first player on the team to bowl. Record their score and then request the first player of the next team to bowl and so on. The amount of support each individual will need will depend upon the activity level they are within and their physical abilities. You can bowl sitting down, but good trunk control and balance are needed. A chair with arms will be helpful, and if this is needed the person should be encouraged to hold on to the arm with their 'non-bowling' hand.

Make sure you give lots of verbal and non-verbal reinforcement of each individual's achieve-ment – urging the ball on, cheering when a skittle is hit, moaning when a skittle does not fall, and shouting 'strike' if all the skittles are knocked down at once.

Monitor the response of the individuals for signs of poor attention, lack of interest or distress. This will help you gauge the pace of the activity and when to end it.

People at the *planned* activity level will enjoy the competitive nature of the game. At the *exploratory* activity level, people will enjoy the process of the game, the running of the ball, the response of their team members. At the *sensory* activity level, you may need to offer the participants hand-over-hand support to facilitate holding and releasing of the ball. The distance between the bowler and skittles will need to be minimal to ensure success and maximum sensory input.

At the end of the activity, thank everyone for participating. Allow for quiet conversation between the participants and encourage them to reflect on the activity.

BEAN-BAG TARGET

This activity can be used to promote the use of physical, social and cognitive skills.

For people who are within the *planned*, *exploratory* or *sensory* activity levels, this activity can be adapted to suit their skills and abilities. Consider the person's:

- personality – do they enjoy social gatherings and physical activity?
- biography – have they played similar games before?
- cognitive ability – is the person able to maintain attention on the game and to follow the rules? Can they let go of the bean bags as they throw them?
- social factors – do they enjoy company? Are there people to whom they seem to relate well?
- physical factors – is the person in a wheelchair? Do they have difficulty with balance and coordination as a result of a stroke or neurological impairment? Do they have arthritis in the joints of their hands that may affect their ability to grip the bean bag?

To play this as a straightforward physical game, unwrap the target and lay it out on a smooth floor, target side up. The pack may already come with bean bags, you may choose to use all or some of them depending on the skills and abilities of the participants. You may purchase bean bags separately and then make your own target. You will need a score board.

The aim of the game is to achieve as high a score as possible by throwing the bean bags one at a time onto the target. The more towards the centre the bean bag lands, the higher the score. If a bean bag lands on the line between two numbers, count the score on which the majority of the bean bag is lying. (Referee's decision is final!)

You may wish to facilitate this activity for a group of four to six individuals. Or you may like to facilitate as a team game, following the guidelines for the ring-toss activity. The person or team that attains the highest score is the winner.

For participants at the *planned* activity level, you can introduce an additional component to the game which will enable participants to use their cognitive skills too. As individuals or within a team, facilitate the activity as described above. After each individual turn, a score is achieved. You can then offer the participants the opportunity to 'double their score' by answering a quiz question. If they answer correctly, the double score is achieved and recorded on the scoreboard. If they answer incorrectly, the original score is recorded.

Your knowledge of the participants will determine the difficulty of the questions asked: too difficult and the participants may feel disheartened, losing interest and attention; too easy and the participants may feel that they are being made fools of and again lose interest.

An additional element can be introduced by asking the participants to choose a category about which they want to answer a question, for example 'food and drink', 'entertainment', 'geography'.

There is a wide variety of quiz books available in book shops; some based on well-known television quizzes, which you may consider a valuable resource when undertaking activities.

For participants at the *exploratory* activity level, the satisfaction will be in the process of the game. Your knowledge of each individual will determine whether you include the quiz element to the game.

Your explanation of the activity will need to be clear and broken down into small steps, perhaps prompting each participant by giving them one bean bag at a time while verbally encouraging and physically demonstrating the throw.

For participants at the *sensory* activity level, the enjoyment of the game will be in the texture of the bean bags in their hands, the sound of the bags hitting the target, the vocalizations of the participants. You may need to offer hand-over-hand support to facilitate hold and release of the bean bags.

At all levels, be mindful of the distance of the target from the participants, giving consideration to their physical skills and needs. For people at a *planned* activity level, the target could be some distance; for those at an *exploratory* activity level, the target may need to be closer; for those at a *sensory* activity level, the target may need to be closer still.

Throughout the game, the facilitation style must be enthusiastic and encouraging. Give lots of verbal and non-verbal feedback and encourage the participants to engage with each other and use their communication skills.

The duration of the game will be guided by the response of the participants. As it finishes, thank everyone for joining in and allow them to sit quietly for a while to reflect and relax.

REFERENCES

Mercer, F. (2006) *Song Book: Words for 100 Popular Songs*. Bicester: Winslow Press.
Music for Dementia: https://m4dradio.com

Chapter 15

CREATIVE ACTIVITIES PACK

SUGGESTED CONTENTS

- Glass pens
- Glass painting cards
- A3 coloured paper
- Paint brushes
- Paint disc set
- Felt-tip pens
- PVA glue
- Collage assortment pack
- Modelling dough
- Modelling set

POSSIBLE SOURCES

Baker Ross Ltd: www.bakerross.co.uk

Hobbycraft: www.hobbycraft.co.uk

NRS Healthcare: www.nrshealthcare.co.uk/health-aids-personal-care/games-craft

Winslow Resources: www.winslowresources.com/rehabilitation-and-functioning/dementia-meaningful-activities.html

The Consortium: www.consortiumeducation.com/care/activities/dementia-activities

INTRODUCTION

Humans have endeavoured to leave their mark on the world since prehistoric times, when the walls of caves were used to record the activities and practices of mankind at that time. Since then, art has been the conduit for the expression of our creative self, for the glorification of gods and rulers, for the recording of historical events, for capturing memories, for pleasure and the innate need to communicate through colour, light and shape.

Whether we are a professional or amateur artist, the satisfaction on completion of something we have created cannot be underestimated, nor can the sense of achievement at the response and recognition of others towards the piece of work. Art is so much more than simply 'putting brush to paper'. The ideas in this activity pack are designed to guide you in facilitating people with cognitive impairments to undertake art/creative activities. You will not be providing art therapy for your clients/service users. In order to offer art therapy, you need to have completed many years of training; indeed, it can be dangerous to attempt to use any therapy techniques unless you have been trained to do so.

The activities described in this pack are designed to be used with people at the *planned*, *exploratory* and *sensory* activity levels.

You will have a good understanding of who is likely to enjoy participating in a creative activity through knowledge of their personality, biography and response to such activities. Do not preclude people who have not undertaken creative activities in the past. This may have been more due to circumstances than choice. Continue to consider people who have a lot of experience in creative arts, indeed who may have been involved professionally. However, be aware of their current skills and abilities compared to what they may have been in the past. Do not place a person in an activity which may reinforce the loss of their skills. Think about presenting creative activities in a different way, but always according to their activity level.

KNOW THE ACTIVITY

You do not need to be a trained artist to be able to facilitate an art or craft activity, but an interest in this type of activity is essential in order to enthuse and engage the participants fully. The following pages provide you with some ideas for the sorts of activities you may like to facilitate.

Ensure that you know what the process of the activity is so that you can assist with problem solving and maintain the focus of the activity. You will need to be fully prepared for the activity and have all the equipment to hand, and check that any co-facilitators understand what is expected of them.

There is a vast range of books and DVDs available in which it may be worth investing.

It is also possible that your local craft store offers classes in particular art or craft activities for facilitators to develop ideas and skills. Perhaps consider a local evening class for yourself and for the person with cognitive impairment. You might also like to consider arranging for an artist or art teacher to offer some classes to facilitators and people with cognitive impairment. Sometimes local art colleges provide sessional input, particularly if it is made part of a student assignment.

(Don't forget about the application of health and safety policies, including the protection of vulnerable adults and the principles of confidentiality, if you do engage people from outside your organization.)

KNOW THE ENVIRONMENT

The facilities and equipment required will obviously depend on the particular activity.

A designated area with table and chairs is ideal, although in some settings you may prefer to use the dining room between meals. The key is that it can be easily cleaned and has access to a sink and water.

Secure storage must be provided for sharp and potentially dangerous tools, as well as toxic materials such as adhesives. There should be relevant completed risk assessments associated with the use and storage of toxic or dangerous materials. Good ventilation, lighting and temperature are essential.

It is extremely important that there is quiet and privacy available to enable participants to fully engage. Distraction and interruption will hinder their ability to focus and concentrate; nobody likes drawing or painting with an audience behind them!

This pack will be appropriate for those who have been established as having ability at either the *planned*, *exploratory* or *sensory* activity level using the QCS Pool Activity Level (PAL) Instrument.

Most of the activities in this pack can be undertaken with an individual on their own or in a small group. Guidance as to the recommended number of participants is given throughout this chapter. Knowledge of the individual, their level of ability, skills, interests, personality and biography, will act as the primary guide for caregivers as to whether to present a creative activity to the individual.

The length of time each activity lasts will be determined by the type of activity and, primarily, by the individual's response to the activity. This relies on the caregiver's observational skills to determine when the activity should cease. People with moderate to severe cognitive impairments may have a very short attention span and the activity may only be appropriate for a very short while.

If safe to do so, some of the activities could be left out for the individual/s to return to when they feel ready. Guidance is given as to the type of activity which could be left out, but a risk assessment for each activity may need to be completed according to the needs of the individuals, the environment and type of service.

UNDERSTANDING THE ABILITY OF THE PERSON

Understanding what a person can and cannot do is vital to the success of the activity. If the activity is too difficult, a person may become anxious or frustrated. If the activity is too easy, the person may feel unmotivated to take part.

Engaging in art and craft activities can provide not only a feeling of personal satisfaction and relaxation during the task, but also a sense of achievement and lasting pleasure in the end result. Of course, art and craft activities are not everyone's 'cup of tea'. Occasionally people may associate some of the activities with school days and be hesitant to engage, according to whether they felt they were 'good at art' or not.

It is also essential that people are not placed in a position where they become aware that they are not as skilled as they used to be in a creative activity, as this can be devastating and lead to the person declining to participate at all.

Consideration at all times must be given to the person's previous experience of creative activities. It is not recommended that someone who was an accomplished artist is given a 'paint by numbers' to complete. This can be very demeaning and negate the skills and life experience of the person. Neither would you ask someone who has no experience of creative activities to undertake a complex craft activity or still-life drawing.

This does not mean that these people cannot be facilitated to engage in a creative activity, however. It is essential that you have a clear understanding of the activity level of the person, so that you know how to present the activity and what sort of activity to offer.

The same issues may need to be considered for the caregivers who will be facilitating a creative activity. Again, some facilitators may have a natural aptitude for creative activities; indeed, it may be a regular pastime for them. Other caregivers may not feel at all confident or interested in creative activities, so ensure that their skills are identified and used in other activities.

Make the most of the 'creative' people in your team, use their skills and ideas.

Planned activity level

At a planned activity level the person can work towards completing a task but may not be able to solve any problems that arise while in the process. They will be able to look in obvious places for objects needed but may not be able to search beyond the usual places. Caregivers assisting someone at this level will need to keep their sentences short and avoid using words like 'and' or 'but' which tend to link two sentences together into a more complex one. Caregivers will also need to stand by to help solve any problems should they arise. People functioning at a planned activity level are able to carry out tasks that achieve a tangible result.

Exploratory activity level

At an exploratory activity level the person can carry out very familiar tasks in familiar surroundings. However, at this level people are more concerned with the effect of doing the activity than in the consequences and may not have an end result in mind. Therefore, a creative and spontaneous approach by caregivers to tasks is helpful. If an activity involves more than two or three tasks, a person at this level will need help in breaking the activity into manageable chunks. Directions need to be made very simple, and the use of memory aids such as task lists, calendars and labelling of frequently used items can be very helpful.

Sensory activity level

At a sensory activity level the person may not have many thoughts or ideas about carrying out an activity; they are mainly concerned with the sensation and with moving their body in response to those sensations. People at this level can be guided to carry out single-step tasks such as sweeping or winding wool. More complex activities can only be carried out when directed one step at a time. Therefore, caregivers need to ensure that the person at this activity level has the opportunity to experience a wide variety of sensations and to carry out one-step tasks. Directions to maximize this opportunity need to be kept very simple and be reinforced by demonstrating the action required.

POTENTIAL BENEFITS OF CREATIVE ACTIVITIES

- May revive a familiar hobby/interest.
- May facilitate learning of a new skill or interest.
- Can improve hand dexterity and coordination.
- Stimulates the senses.
- Facilitates decision-making skills.
- Stimulates the imagination.
- Enables people to experience a sense of achievement.
- Facilitates communication.
- Facilitates reminiscence and orientation.
- Can place someone in the role of expert.

Before embarking on these activities, consider the person's:

- personality – is the person motivated to take part? Are they interested in art/craft? Does the person have an awareness that their level of skill in this activity may not be as good as it was? This will have a huge effect on the person's sense of self and confidence. How will the person view the activity? You will need to ensure that you present it in an appropriate manner so participants do not feel that the activity is childish or that they are being treated like children. Would the person be active or passive during the activity?

- biography – does the person have good memories of this activity which will enhance their confidence and self-esteem, or do they have negative memories associated with this activity which may be painful for them?

- cognitive ability – do you know for how long each person is able to concentrate? Does each person require very specific, simple, one-step instructions to be able to participate? Does the person understand what is being asked of them? Do they comprehend the purpose of the activity or are they more likely to enjoy the sensation of the activity? Is the person able to solve problems if required? Does the person have intact visual recognition skills for all the objects used? Is the person able to use their memory to remember familiar skills and actions? Is the person able to express their preferences, choices and wishes? Does the person have a sense of control over their environment and activities and opportunities?

- social factors – do they enjoy company? Are there people to whom they seem to relate well? Is the person able to express their emotions? (Art may be a useful technique for expression in the absence of words.) Would the person prefer to engage in the activity on their own or in a small group? What is the person's preferred communication method? Do they use a variety of communication techniques, verbal and non-verbal, or do they have difficulties with communication? Does the person enjoy being with others? Are they able to understand functions such as sharing and turn taking?

- physical factors – is the person able to sit for the duration of an activity? Do they require the seating to be at a certain height and are they able to tolerate sitting in a straight-backed, firm chair? Does the person have a good range of movement? Are they able to reach items required? Can they utilize all of the paper or does it need to be made smaller? Does the person have good dexterity and coordination? Can they hold a paint brush or pencil, or would they benefit from an adaptation to the brush or pencil? Does the person have arthritic pain, stiffness to the joints? Does the person have a neurological impairment – such as a tremor or a weakness to one side of their body or a paralysis – affecting their physical ability and requiring support? (An occupational therapist will be able to advise you on how to support people with these difficulties to participate in an art activity.)

WHAT ARE THE SENSORY NEEDS OF THE PERSON?

Does the person have a visual impairment? Can they see strong, primary colours and patterns? Does the person wear glasses and are these clean? Can they see the edge of the paper or card; is there a contrasting colour underneath? Does the person have a hearing impairment; do they need to be able to hear instructions in order to participate in the activity? Do they wear a hearing aid, and is it switched on? Is the person able to use their other senses, for example touch for craft-type activities, feeling texture and shape and using hands as a paint brush?

Could you enhance the experience of the person by engaging their sense of smell, perhaps very aromatic flowers, spices or fruits?

GLASS PAINTING CARDS AND GLASS PENS

Cards are available in a range of themes, including religious festivals, birthdays or anniversaries. This activity will be extremely useful in providing assistive cues in orientating the person with cognitive impairment to the time of year.

The sending of Christmas cards, for example, has been an essential part of the celebration of Christmas since Victorian times. Many people are likely to have a strong memory for this activity and may recall the feelings associated with the giving and receiving of cards.

It is equally likely that the person will have some experience of making greetings cards, either as a child or adult, or of helping children to make cards. There is an understanding, too, that receiving a handmade card is something extra special in recognition of the thought, time and effort put into this.

People who enjoy art and craft will enjoy this activity because it involves elements of both pastimes.

The activity of glass painting cards is designed to be carried out with people at the *planned* and *exploratory* activity levels.

Packs vary depending on the source, but typically consist of:

- card templates
- acetates each with pictures etched onto them
- glass pens/markers.

Instructions for completing a card

1. Choose a picture and cut along the outer edge (where indicated) to remove from the sheet.
2. Using glass pens, colour in the picture, remaining within the black lines.
3. Choose a card and remove the detachable outer edge and detachable oblong of card where the picture will go.
4. Fold the card at the indentation.
5. Remove the white tissue backing from the picture on the acetate.
6. Carefully place the picture behind the oblong hole on the front of the card. Ensure that the coloured surface is facing outward.
7. Using double-sided clear tape, or glue which dries clear, attach the picture to the inside of the card.
8. You may like to use some glitter or glitter pens to decorate the outer edge of the card.

Presentation of this activity to a person at the planned activity level

A person at the *planned* activity level will very much enjoy this activity in terms of working towards a tangible end result. The steps for completion of the greetings card are clearly defined and very straightforward and the person is likely to require minimum prompting to complete each step. Though the steps for completion of the card are defined, there is room for personal creativity in terms of choice of the picture and colours used to complete it and choice of card in which to stick the picture.

When facilitating a person to engage in this activity, it may be a good idea to have a completed card to show them in order to enable them to envisage what the end result will be and what can be achieved. (The 'here's one I made earlier' technique is very useful.)

Be mindful that the pictures are simple and may be construed as quite childlike. People may associate the idea of 'colouring in' as a childhood pursuit. However, people can be encouraged to participate in terms of the simplicity of the cards; the process of 'colouring in' can be very relaxing and provide stimulation for the senses. This activity also promotes choice and decision-making skills.

A group of people at the planned activity level may wish to engage in this activity together, either as a group of individuals or as a team. Perhaps forming a production line where different steps in the process are undertaken by different people would be fun, one person cutting out the pictures, one or two colouring them, one sticking them on the card, one or two people decorating the cards, and so on. Make sure that you provide an opportunity for everyone to undertake each step of the activity at some point.

This will be highly motivating for the participants who will be using not only their creative and cognitive skills, but also their communication and social skills.

The activity also assists people at the planned activity level as all the objects needed are in front of them; they do not need to search for them.

Facilitators for this activity need to ensure that they fully prepare and organize the activity in advance:

- Identify an area where there will be no distractions or interruptions, if possible.
- Ensure that the room is well lit and that the temperature is appropriate. There will need to be a source of ventilation as the glass pens have a strong smell.
- Prepare the table and ensure that all the equipment you need is there.
- Make sure that there are enough comfortable seats for everyone.
- Be prepared to offer advice, support and prompting as required.
- Give praise and reinforcement throughout.
- Consider what is to be done with the completed cards. Will the participants keep them, could they be sold, if appropriate, as a contribution to the service's funds? Involve the participants in this decision.

Presentation of this activity to a person at the exploratory activity level

A person at the *exploratory* activity level will enjoy this activity because of its familiarity and opportunity to be creative. People at this activity level will enjoy the process of the craft, the stimulation of the senses and the opportunity for social engagement. They are likely to be less concerned with the end result.

You can use the same techniques for engaging, preparing and facilitating as detailed above. Be mindful of the skills and abilities of each individual in terms of dexterity, attention and concentration, and problem solving. They may require more intense support and guidance from facilitators to enable them to remain focused and to gain a sense of pleasure and achievement.

Accuracy may not be as important as the taking part for this group of individuals, therefore be careful that you do not refer to errors in a negative way or attempt to correct errors unless requested to, as this will have a negative impact on the participants' sense of well-being and motivation to participate.

Collaboration of participants and facilitators in this activity is essential and great fun!

On completion of this activity, thank all the participants for their contribution and for joining in. Allow time for reflection, perhaps by looking at the completed cards and talking about them, favourite colours, designs and so on. Encourage participants to reminisce about the season, perhaps enjoy a cup of tea together while doing so. Some participants may like to assist you in clearing up after the activity.

Additional ideas

If participants have enjoyed this activity, they may like to continue glass painting as a club. Glass paints and pens are readily available from most craft shops and some stationers. You could save and collect a store of jam jars and glass bottles for people to paint. You will need a black glass marker to draw the design on the glass first. Enable participants to be spontaneous and creative using abstract and representational designs.

You could also try painting on glass sheets. The process is quite simple. Encourage participants to choose a picture, perhaps from a magazine, and trace over it with tracing paper using a black felt-tip pen. Place the tracing under a sheet of A4 glass. Using a glass pen or marker, follow the tracing underneath so that the picture is replicated onto the glass, then remove the tracing paper from underneath and colour in the drawing using glass paints or pens. Consider framing the pictures by placing a piece of black card behind the finished picture and installing in a suitable frame.

People may like to paint their own designs directly onto the glass.

WARNING

Glass pens/markers are spirit based. Ensure that these are not ingested and are used in a well-ventilated room. They may stain skin and clothes.

Refer to manufacturer for guidance.

Be cautious in the use of glass and guard against breakage and possible cuts. You may consider undertaking a risk assessment of the activity and individuals to inform you as to how to proceed or reduce the risks identified.

ART/CREATIVE ACTIVITIES USING PAPER, PAINT AND FELT-TIP PENS

For people at the planned activity level

A regular 'art' group, perhaps once a week, may be of great interest and very motivating for people. You can decide the theme of each session together in advance. The group members may wish to concentrate on their own work or participate in a group piece. Suggested themes:

- still-life work, such as fruit, vegetables, interesting objects, flowers
- architecture and buildings
- landscape
- self-portrait
- people
- animals
- the seasons

- view from a window.

Be mindful of different levels of artistic ability within the group, particularly if you are sharing the work. Some people may wish to keep their work private. Respect this. You may consider working from photographs or pictures. Facilitate this by reinforcing the link between the photo and the painting or drawing to enable participants to remain focused. Make sure the photo is big enough for them to see.

Consult with the participants about what they wish to be done with the completed work. Are there opportunities for framing work? Would the group consider an art exhibition once or twice a year?

GREETINGS CARDS

It may be possible that people will enjoy using their art work to make greetings cards. You may need to frame their work in strong card so that it is more substantial. Again, craft shops have an array of pictures, printing tools, transfers and materials specifically for card making.

IMAGINATION

Make use of a person's imagination, playfulness and creativity. Encourage participants to paint from their imagination or perhaps a cherished memory. Facilitate this process by writing down the person's ideas to help their recall and to maintain focus on the picture.

ABSTRACT DESIGNS

The paint and paper could also be used for printing a design or abstract image. Ensure that the person's clothing is protected. Have a variety of fruits, vegetables, leaves, flowers suitable for printing with, for example half an apple, a piece of carrot cut crossways, an oak leaf – anything hard (that will withstand paint and pressure) and with an interesting design. Cover the surface to be printed in paint and place down firmly on paper for a few seconds. Carefully lift the object off. Repeat. Allow the prints to dry. These can be used as background for other pieces of work if desired.

Use the paper and paint, pens and so on for abstract work emphasizing pattern, design and flow of ideas. This may be a difficult concept for some participants who may be more conscious of concrete ideas and 'recognizable' art. It may be useful to have ideas and pictures for them to see and perhaps copy, using a colour of their choice.

CREATIVE WRITING

Rather than using the paper and pens for drawing, consider using them for creative writing. This is particularly good in a small group. Agree what you would like to write about. Enable the participants to choose colours and write their ideas, according to the topic, on the paper. This may be a little daunting for some participants, in which case a better idea is for the facilitator to write down what the group members say according to the topic and colour choices. This takes great concentration by the facilitator, who must write down what the participants say, not their interpretation of what is said.

Suggested topics:

- The seasons, using colour to represent each of the different seasons
- The weather, again using colour to represent the different types
- Holidays, using colour to represent different countries, beaches
- Special occasions

- The countryside.

Some people may like to complete their own piece of writing or use a combination of picture and writing to express a particular theme or idea.

For people at the exploratory activity level

This group of people are likely to enjoy the process of the activity, being less concerned with the end result. They will enjoy the opportunity to use and explore colours, shapes and designs. With some encouragement, they may be stimulated by the other members of the group and engage in conversation about what they are doing or of what it reminds them of. People at the *exploratory* activity level may not be able to concentrate for too long at a time, so consider artistic activities that have fairly quick results.

SIMPLE SCENES

Participants may enjoy completing a skyscape or a seascape. This can be achieved quite quickly by using broad, sweeping strokes, with the paint brush loaded with paint, across the paper. The participants may require guidance as to the choice of colours, perhaps blues and greens for sea and sky, reds and yellows for sunset. Have some examples or photographs to inspire them.

PAINTING TO MUSIC

This is a very enjoyable and relaxing activity. You will need to prepare a variety of musical styles, but may wish to concentrate on relaxing tunes: the classics or 'chilled' playlists. Inform the participants that they will be using their imagination and allowing their arm and the paint brush or pen to move as though it is 'dancing to the music'. Play some music to engage the attention and then ask the participants to paint or draw whatever comes to mind or just to move their arm across the paper in time to the music. You may need to demonstrate this activity first. There may be a variety of results, representational and abstract.

STRING PAINTING

You may like to engage the participants in another kind of printing technique. Fold a piece of paper in half. Dip a long piece of string in paint and lay it over one half of the paper in a random design. Close the other half of the paper over it and press down hard. If there is an end of the piece of string hanging out between the folded paper, pull it out *without* opening the paper. Once the string is removed, open the paper to see the results!

Note, any kind of technique which has an element of surprise will be very motivating and engaging for people at the *exploratory* (and *sensory*) activity level. Another idea is to again fold a piece of paper in half. On one side of the paper use lots of paint to make an abstract design; the design should touch the fold of the paper but not go over it. When the person is satisfied with the design, fold the paper in half over the design and press gently. Do not rub the design as this will result in a mucky splodge! Carefully unfold the paper and admire the results.

These techniques are somewhat messy. Be guided by the response of the participants as to whether they feel comfortable with this and ensure that clothing is protected.

ART CORNER

Do not underestimate the artistic skills of people at the exploratory activity level. Encourage people to use these skills by setting up an 'art corner' for them or ensuring that there are art materials readily available to them, to make use of moments of spontaneity.

People at this activity level will also enjoy creative writing, particularly if they do not need to do the writing! This is a marvellous opportunity for social interaction and reminiscence, recorded for posterity, and a chance to be creative with words. The fact that it is being recorded on a large piece of paper in bright colours will enable the participants to maintain focus on the activity and enjoy the process.

For people at the *sensory* activity level, you may wish to facilitate someone in a one-to-one art activity to enable them to experience as much sensory stimulation as possible. A person at the *sensory* activity level will not be concerned with the outcome of the activity or necessarily the process. What they will enjoy are the colours, shapes, textures and sounds that you can introduce into an art activity.

The individual activities do not have to last a long time; a fairly immediate result will be very motivating for the individual whose concentration skills may be quite limited.

GUIDED COLOURING

The person may respond to stark, contrast images of no more than two colours. Having a pre-drawn outline on a large piece of paper for the person to paint is one idea. The outline could be of a face in silhouette or an animal or a familiar object. You will need to guide the person, perhaps using hand-over-hand, to dip a large, thick brush into the paint and place it on the paper. Use broad sweeping strokes to enable the person to experience the sensation of movement.

You can use the same idea for painting flowers. Use a whole piece of paper and a black pen to draw a huge flower (not too complex). Facilitate the person to paint the petals, leaves and stem in colours of their choice. Use any object or theme of particular interest or relevance to the person.

Be mindful of visual impairment and cognitive impairment. The person's world may be quite small to them, so you may wish to try this technique on a piece of A4 paper to enable the person to focus on it a little easier.

Again, the outcome is not of importance here. It is the person's *sensory* experience of the activity which is important.

HAND PAINTING

Some people may enjoy a very simple printing technique – brushing paint over the hand, placing it firmly on paper and removing it to reveal a print. Feet are sometimes fun to print with, too.

If you are hoping to engage a person at the *sensory* activity level in this activity, be very mindful of the potential risks and comfort of the person. Your knowledge of the person will enable you to decide whether this would be enjoyable for them. By constantly monitoring their verbal and non-verbal responses, you will know whether to proceed with the activity.

By its nature, this is a messy activity. Be conscious of protecting clothing and assisting the individuals not to put their hands in their mouths until all paint traces have been removed.

People at the *sensory* activity level may also enjoy painting to music. The sound of the music, the bright colours and sweeping movements of the hand will be stimulating. Again, you may wish to offer hand-over-hand assistance to enable the person to participate in the activity.

DOOR NAMEPLATES

Personalized bedroom doors can help individuals to identify their own rooms. This can be achieved through colour, door furniture and a nameplate placed in a picture frame at eye level on the door. If the person is involved in the creation of the nameplate, it is likely to be easier to identify. This is a very simple and straightforward activity which someone can do on their own or as part of a small group.

People who are at the *planned* or *exploratory* activity level can be helped as described below. Those with less ability will need more help and support from an activity worker, key worker, relative or care worker.

You will need to supply thin card in a range of colours, a variety of paints, pencils, felt-tip and marker pens, scissors and PVA glue.

When inviting people to participate in this activity with you, it may be useful for you to have a completed door nameplate to show them to enable them to understand what you are asking them to do.

Each participant will be asked to pick a background card according to their colour preference. Invite them to write their name on it or perhaps a name by which they are usually known or prefer to be called. Encourage this to be done in a size large enough to be read from a distance. You could draw a set of parallel lines on the card to facilitate this. Enable the person to decide what coloured medium they would like to use – a mixture of paint and pen is entirely acceptable. You may need to guide the person to write their name. Make sure that the paint or pen is completely dry before giving the nameplate to the person. Better still, if you are in a residential establishment, take the person and the nameplate to their room to enable them to fully complete the activity. (This may be particularly important for people at the planned activity level who may be very concerned with the outcome of the activity and would value the opportunity to see it through from beginning to end.)

Added extras...

- Encourage the participants to add pictures by drawing or painting.
- Perhaps add a photograph of the person.
- Have some magazines available and facilitate the person to choose favourite pictures to stick on the nameplate.
- Use stickers readily available from craft shops to add to the nameplate.
- Consider using glitter and metallic pens for that extra bit of 'bling'.

The person may not wish to put their name on the door, so consider options such as 'Do not disturb', 'Quiet please', 'Please knock before entering' or any message the person would like to write.

People at the *exploratory* activity level will enjoy the process of the activity but may not recollect that the nameplate is for their door. People at the *planned* activity level will look forward to the outcome as long as they are happy with their completed nameplate.

In either case, if the person does not wish to use their nameplate, do not force them to.

COLLAGE ASSORTMENT PACK AND PVA GLUE

The items in the collage assortment box should be a cacophony of colour, texture and light. You can buy ready-made packs from sources such as the ones at the start of this chapter, or you can build your own collection. No one could fail to be thrilled and enticed by the glamour of the sequins, the sparkle of the pipe cleaners and ribbons, the fantasy of the feathers.

One gazes into the box with an almost childlike excitement and yearning to feel the items inside. Boxes like this engage the sense of wonder and playfulness in all humans – no matter what the age. This impact alone is reason enough to share the box with the people for whom you care. We are never too old to imagine or to create. People with cognitive impairments are no less able to call on these skills and concepts, and with careful facilitation can enter a new world of excitement and fantasy.

Unfortunately, collage work has long been associated with either school days or older people sitting around a table with a few odd bits of material and magazines, wishing they were somewhere else. The box in this activity pack gives you the opportunity to provide a very different experience of collage work. The skills and opportunities this activity provides for people with cognitive impairments are not only about creativity, but also sharing, communication and teamwork.

For people at the *planned* and *exploratory* activity levels, working on a collage which they have designed and contributed to can be an extremely pleasurable and stimulating experience. Items in this pack will also be of interest to people at a *sensory* or a *reflex* activity level.

By understanding the skills, abilities and preferences of the people for whom you care, you will be able to identify who would most enjoy participating in this activity. It is important not to mix people from different activity levels. Those at the *planned* activity level will be very determined about the finished product: what it should look like, where different materials should go and so on. People at the *exploratory* activity level are likely to be less concerned with the outcome, enjoying the process more. This could lead to some tension within the group, particularly if problems arise, which may be difficult for the participants to manage. As facilitator, you need to monitor the response of each individual group member to ensure that they are enjoying the activity and that they receive recognition for their skills and contribution to the activity. You will need to support participants through any differences of opinion regarding completion of the activity, ensuring that everyone has an opportunity to participate, though some clear leaders may emerge in the group.

If one of the participants has particular expertise in this type of activity, involve them as co-facilitator to maximize opportunities to build their self-esteem.

The running of the group

Make sure that you have an allocated space or a room in which to hold the activity. This needs to be free of interruptions, well lit and well ventilated. It is important to consider the skills and expertise of the individuals involved in the activity when deciding how many people to invite into the group. You can do this with just one person, of course, and no more than six people would be the optimum.

When inviting participants into the group, it may be useful to have a completed collage or picture to show them, or to take the box of collage materials to entice them!

The room must be fully prepared for the group's arrival. You will need:

- a table and chairs
- a protective cover for the table, for example a large piece of plastic sheeting
- large pieces of card which can be taped together once the group has decided how big the collage will be
- the collage box which contains folds of metallic material, feathers, glitter pipe cleaners, sequin mesh and sequin rows, ribbons, gold and silver braid, holographic and metallic card and paper
- PVA glue, decanted into small pots or trays (one for each participant), and a glue brush for each participant

- scissors – being mindful of any associated risks.

Additional items which you may wish to provide include:

- a selection of magazines, postcards and used greetings cards
- textural items such as cotton wool, string, egg boxes, leaves, dried flower heads, thistles
- anything which would orientate the group to the season.

Welcome the participants into the group and explain what they will be doing. Share some pictures to enable the group members to begin to identify a theme for their collage.

Suggested themes

- Underwater fantasy
- A day at the seaside
- Holidays
- Countryside
- The seasons
- Theatre night
- Fashion
- Food, glorious food!
- Industry
- Religious festivals
- High days and holidays
- Favourite things
- Weather
- Light and dark
- Historical events (according to time of year in which the anniversary is celebrated)
- Science fiction fantasy

Once the group has chosen a theme, decide how big the collage will be and adapt your paper or card accordingly. You may wish to complete a rough sketch on the paper, with guidance from the group, as to the positioning of elements of the collage – for example, sea and sky, land, buildings, trees.

Enable the group to explore all the different materials available. Some decisions will begin to be made about which materials would suit which element of the collage. Put the materials on the rough design according to where they will be positioned in the final collage.

You may like to allocate specific tasks to the individual group members, with their agreement. This will be particularly helpful to people at the *planned* activity level, who will appreciate clearly identified tasks which they can complete before moving on to the next task. People at the *exploratory* activity level will enjoy one-step tasks, but may require additional support and guidance to maintain focus and momentum.

Suggested tasks

- Collecting suitable materials, for example of the same colour/texture.
- Cutting chosen material into shapes.

- Gluing material onto the collage.
- Working on a specific element of the collage, for example sky, sea, figures.
- Working on a specific area of the collage, for example bottom/top corner, left/right side.
- Overseeing the whole collage, keeping people on track, keeping an image of the finished collage in mind, referring to the original picture if one is being used as a guide.

Play some gentle music, related to the theme if possible, in the background as people work. Encourage interaction and sharing, decision making, reminiscence and laughter. Constantly monitor the response of the individuals. Have a tea or coffee break at an appropriate moment and allow the participants to reflect on the work so far.

You will need to decide whether the collage has to be finished in one session. Can you arrange another session with the participants? Can you leave it out safely for participants to work on at their leisure? Do you have somewhere you can store the 'work in progress' and all the materials? Make sure that you have safely disposed of any glue which has not been used.

Always thank the participants for joining in with the activity and for their contribution. Specifically highlight one thing for each individual which has impressed you and tell them so, as part of the group reflection. Ask the group participants what they have enjoyed.

Ultimately decide with the participants where the collage will be hung. An unveiling ceremony might be fun, if the 'collage makers' are in agreement.

More ideas...

You could facilitate individuals to complete their own collage. Enable them to choose the size of paper to work on; A4 may be suitable. They can choose their materials and theme and work on this independently or among a group of others who are all working on their own collages.

The collages could remain individual or the participants may agree for them to be stuck together, particularly if they are all on the same theme.

People at the *sensory* activity level might enjoy the collage pack in a different way. They may be able to contribute to the completion of the collage, given verbal and physical guidance on a one-to-one basis throughout. They may, more simply, enjoy exploring the contents of the box, feeling the different textures and seeing the different colours and sparkle. This relates well to the sort of sensory work which really stimulates people at this activity level.

You could also select specific items from the box that have an interesting texture, a strong colour or some sparkle and share them, one at a time, with people at a *reflex* activity level. Some lurex material placed in the palm of the hand may elicit a grasp response, or a feather in a bright colour stroked on the back of the hand may be of interest to the person.

It is essential that the collage facilitators are enthusiastic about this activity and have some skill themselves. This will help to generate ideas and identify the process, contributing significantly to the design. If you have access to the internet there are some fascinating websites specifically on collage and ideas. Type 'collage ideas' into your search engine.

MODELLING DOUGH AND MODELLING SET

Creativity and art is all about stimulating the senses and freeing the mind. Mankind has used sculpture as an artistic medium for thousands of years, again in veneration of deities, recording of historical events and expression of the self. As children, we often enjoyed the tactile sensation of clay and play doh and the myriad forms we could make from it. As we grew older, we used clay and other pliable materials to make three-dimensional figures or things we could use such as mugs, boxes, badges, jewellery. A gift which someone has made is always a delight to receive. For some, this enjoyment has become a much-loved hobby or a business.

Whether for play or for profit, using and modelling clay or dough enables us to use and develop a variety of skills which are transferable; for example, modelling dough can be replaced with pastry dough.

These are some of the benefits of using modelling dough with people with cognitive impairments:

- Places emphasis on use of the senses, particularly touch and vision.
- Provides a straightforward series of single steps to achieve an outcome.
- Gives quick results to engage concentration and attention skills.
- Enables familiar patterns of movement to be elicited.
- Evokes memories that can lead to reminiscence.
- Provides opportunities to learn or re-establish a skill.
- Provides opportunities for communication and social interaction – verbal and non-verbal.
- Exercises joints and muscles of hands.
- Facilitates use of imagination and play.
- Enables errors to be turned into successes quickly and easily.
- Provides opportunities to experience a sense of achievement.
- Provides opportunities to transfer skills learned in other types of activity, such as baking.

Be careful to present this activity appropriately so that people do not feel that you are treating them childishly.

People at the *planned* activity level may enjoy modelling the dough, being conscious of complex uses for it with definite end results in mind: figurines, models of animals and so on. They may wish to use the different coloured doughs on a single piece (e.g. modelling a bowl of fruit or bunch of flowers). This may lead them on to modelling with air-hardening dough or salt dough to achieve a more lasting result. The modelling dough can be used for people at the *exploratory* and *sensory* activity levels. What is most engaging about this activity is the effect on the senses, which will be really motivating for the participants. The colours are bright, the dough smells wonderful and the feel of it as it is moulded in the hands is relaxing and soothing.

One of the aims of this activity is to enable people to use choice: to pick the colour dough with which they want to work, to mould an object of their choice or just to handle the dough. People may not have an idea of what they want to mould until they actually start handling the dough. For people at these activity levels it is not necessary to pursue an 'end result', though they might surprise themselves with a skill they did not know they had!

Enable participants to handle the dough and use the modelling set too. The modelling set typically consists of rolling pins, spatulas and a variety of dough cutters. You can buy these as sets or obtain items individually.

Facilitate the participants to use some of these items to explore the dough even more.

People at the *sensory* activity level may need hand-over-hand assistance to do this. Constantly monitor the response of the participants, to ensure that they are enjoying the activity and sensation of the dough in their hands. Once finished with, the dough can be remoulded and shaped back into tubes to be placed in the plastic bags for use next time. Try to ensure that mixed colours of dough are taken apart before remoulding.

Be conscious of whether the person would like to keep the object they have made.

PRECAUTIONS

Please be advised that the colour on the dough does come off on the hands. This is easily washed off with soap and water. You will need to consider protecting clothes in case someone rubs their hands over them, but again the colour will wash out.

Be aware that people may take the dough to their mouths and may try to eat it. Please support participants to prevent this from happening as part of your risk assessment of the person and activity. The dough is non-toxic, but if some is eaten, you may wish to seek medical advice.

SUMMARY

Art activities provide a wonderful way to enable people at all activity levels to express themselves, and they should be good fun too.

You will always be guided by the needs, preferences and responses of the individuals with whom you are working. Facilitators are required to be knowledgeable and enthusiastic, too, to really maximize opportunities for engagement and a sense of purpose.

Be mindful always of how you present the activity in order that it meets the activity level of the person *now*, not what it may have been some years ago. Also be aware of how you assess and manage the risks associated with using paint and coloured pens.

Lastly, always be encouraging, reassuring and supportive. A facilitator's role is not to criticize, not to 'correct', not to pass judgement. It is to facilitate, enable and empower.

Chapter 16

SENSORY ACTIVITIES PACK

SUGGESTED CONTENTS

- Relaxation music playlist
- Rainmaker
- Doll or HUG™
- Foot spa
- Coloured light sphere lamp
- Vibrating pillow
- Bumpie ball
- Lavender moisturizing body lotion

POSSIBLE SOURCES

HUG™: www.hug.world

ROMPA: www.rompa.com/catalogsearch/result/?q=dementia

TFH Special Needs Toys: https://specialneedstoys.com/uk/search?query=dementia

INTRODUCTION

This pack will be appropriate for those at *sensory* and *reflex* activity levels of ability using the QCS Pool Activity Level (PAL) Instrument. However, individuals at a *planned* and an *exploratory* activity level may also enjoy and benefit from these sensory experiences.

Most of the objects in this pack are intended to be used in individual activity sessions with the carer. It is possible that some may also be used in a small group, but the carer will need to observe each participant and judge if all are gaining something from the activity. The length of time each activity lasts will, again, be determined by the individual's response to the object, and will rely on the carer's observational skills to determine when the activity should cease. People with moderate to severe cognitive impairments may have a very short attention span and the activity may only be appropriate for a few minutes. In these cases, it is best to use a 'little and often' approach.

UNDERSTANDING THE ABILITY OF THE PERSON

Understanding what the person can and cannot do is vital to the success of the activity. If an activity is too difficult, a person may become anxious or frustrated. If the activity is too easy, the person may not feel motivated to take part.

A person who has moderate to severe impairments is likely to be responding to their world mainly through the senses, even in a purely reflex response to specific stimuli. When we know this, we can help the person to engage with their world by presenting sensations to the person. Therefore, some of the activities in this pack are particularly beneficial for people at a *sensory* or a *reflex* activity level.

Sensory activity level

At a *sensory* activity level, the person may not have many thoughts or ideas about carrying out an activity; they are mainly concerned with the sensation and with moving their body in response to those sensations. People at this level can be guided to carry out single-step tasks such as sweeping or winding wool. More complex activities can only be carried out when directed one step at a time. Caregivers therefore need to ensure that the person at this activity level has the opportunity to experience a wide variety of sensations, and to carry out one-step tasks. Directions to maximize this opportunity need to be kept very simple and to be reinforced by demonstrating the action required.

Reflex activity level

A person at a *reflex* activity level may not be aware of the surrounding environment or even of their own body. They are living in a subliminal or sub-conscious state, where movement is a reflex response to a stimulus. Therefore, people wishing to enter into this person's consciousness need to use direct sensory stimulation. By using direct stimulation, the person's self-awareness can be raised. A person at this level may have difficulty in processing more than one sensation at a time. Excessive or multiple stimuli can cause distress, so crowds, loud noises and background clamour should be avoided. Activities at this level should focus on introducing a single sensation to the person. A caregiver interacting with a person at a *reflex* activity level needs to use all their communication skills to enter into the person's world at their level. Language skills tend to play only a minor role at this level and should be kept to single words, although the use of facial expression and of a warm and reassuring tone and volume can be vital in establishing a communication channel.

RELAXATION MUSIC

Music is a very personal choice, but it touches most of us with its ability to enhance mood and well-being. The rhythm and beat of music can have a direct effect on the physical functions of the body; a slow rhythm influences the heart to beat more slowly and leads to a sense of calm and relaxation. There are many playlists of this type on music-streaming devices.

There are several ways that this music might be used. It may form the end of a more invigorating activity, such as a group game or a 'movement to music' session that encourages mobility. Some ideas for this are presented below. Alternatively, the music may be used simply as a relaxation activity in a group or individually for people who need help to relax.

Relaxation technique

Make sure that everyone is sitting comfortably; that their heads and arms are supported and that their feet are firmly on the floor.

For people who are able to imitate movement and to follow instructions (*sensory*, *exploratory* and *planned* activity levels), demonstrate the following actions and encourage them to copy you. Reinforce people's involvement with smiles and nods.

- Tighten the muscles in your toes. Hold for a count of 10. Relax and enjoy the sensation of release from tension.
- Flex the muscles in your feet. Hold for a count of 10. Relax.
- Move slowly up through your body – legs, abdomen, back, neck, face – contracting and relaxing muscles as you go.
- Now close your eyes and listen to the music while you breathe deeply and slowly.
- Finally, stop the music, ask everyone to open their eyes and encourage them to gently stretch and to look around them.
- Thank everyone for joining in and ask if they would like to do the activity again at another time.

You will need to make more direct contact with people who are unable to imitate movement and to follow instructions (*reflex* activity level). This is likely to be a one-to-one activity. Sit next to and slightly to one side of the person and gently and firmly hold their hands. Make eye contact, smile and nod, and say 'listen' and 'lovely' and breathe deeply. Stroke the back of the person's hand, using firm and gentle movements that are in time with the beat of the music.

Movement to music

Select music with a strong, fairly fast beat. Make sure people who are at risk of falling are seated. Hand out two brightly coloured scarves to each person and keep two for yourself. Begin to wave them in time to the music and encourage others to join in. Play two fast tunes.

Now play the relaxation music and encourage everyone to listen to it and to relax.

Variations

- Use a large cloth or parachute and ask everyone to hold on to it. This forms a connection with each other, and may be useful for people who are more impaired (*reflex* activity level) and need more help to make movements.
- For people who can imitate the actions of another person (*sensory*, *exploratory* or *planned* activity levels), lead everyone to move different parts of the body, starting with the shoulders:
    - shoulders: shrugging and relaxing
    - arms: straight out in front and moving to the side and back straight out in front and raising up and down out to each side and turning small circles
    - hands: miming playing the piano, turning the wrists and hands over and back
    - waist: leaning forwards while holding onto the chair arms, turning to the left and then to the right
    - legs: stamping feet up and down
    - knees: straightening and bending
    - ankles: pointing feet to the ceiling and down to the floor, drawing circles with the toes.

RAINMAKER

The traditional rainsticks originated in northern Chile where they are used in ceremonies to bring rain. They are made from the skeleton of the capado cactus – when the cactus dies it is dried, hollowed out and filled with small seeds or pebbles. Small nails are driven through the hull of the cactus in a spiral formation, and when the rainstick is inverted the filling strikes the nails, creating the sound of falling water. Commercially available rainmakers come in a variety of sizes, materials and colours, from plastic ones filled with brightly coloured beads to wooden ones. All are designed to enable users to enjoy watching, hearing and feeling the 'rain' fall. By holding it straight up and down or angled, you can create anything from a hurricane to a gentle spring shower. Plastic rainmakers have special prisms in the walls of the instrument to create a rainbow of colours as the beads cascade through the tube. Those with a rubber ring exterior help to give an easy grip when used.

The rainmaker is intended for use by people with severe cognitive impairments (*reflex* activity level) who will be engaging with their world through the senses of touch, hearing and sight. It can help the person to focus on an object and to sustain their attention for a few moments.

Show the person the rainmaker and invert it to reveal how it works. Use smiles and nods and say 'listen' and 'look' to show the person what is happening.

Offer the rainmaker to the person. Help them to hold and move it (you may need to hold your hand over the person's).

This may be an activity of only a few moments. Carefully observe the response of the person by looking at their body language, particularly facial expression and posture. Remove the rainmaker if the person responds negatively to it or begins to lose interest.

Leave the rainmaker with the person if they engage positively with it. If the person takes the rainmaker to their mouth to explore it, encourage this to happen. Clean the rainmaker afterwards with a mild antibacterial solution.

Finish by thanking the person for taking part (even if the person does not seem to know what you are saying, the tone of your voice will be important).

DOLLS

Dolls have long been recognized as an integral part of human development and play throughout the centuries and across cultures. Children have longed for the 'doll of the year' at Christmas time and adult collectors have searched for the exquisite 'limited edition doll'.

When we are working with people with cognitive impairment the use of dolls provides us with the opportunity to explore the many facets of a human being in terms of emotional expression, communication, attachment, development and playfulness.

Therapeutic dolls are commercially available. You may wish to dress the doll or have a variety of clothing available for it.

HUG™ is a highly therapeutic doll-like sensory product designed to be cuddled. It has a beating heart within its soft body and can play music from a favourite playlist. HUG™ also comes with a set of guides that describe how to use it with people at each of the PAL levels.

For people who have moderate to severe cognitive impairments (sensory and reflex activity levels), the doll or HUG™ may be used to assist in the enhancement of well-being as well as to provide an opportunity for the person to engage in meaningful interaction, expression of emotion and demonstration of the role of 'mother' or 'father'.

It is not always necessary or appropriate to directly give a person the doll in the first instance. Place the doll within the visual field of the person and use verbal, non-verbal and sensory cues to direct the person towards the doll. The cue may be the texture of the doll's garment or skin, the colour of the garment or the smell (rub a little baby powder on to the doll).

Carefully monitor the person's response, particularly their facial expression. The person may smile at the doll or reach out for it. If this happens, place the doll on the person's lap or in the cradle of the person's elbow.

Continue to closely monitor the response of the person. They may rock the doll, speak to it or sing. If the person is singing, join in gently and quietly. Encourage the person to stroke the doll. The person may wish to play with the doll's garments, or remove them. Again, join in with positive verbal and non-verbal responses, constantly monitoring the response of the person.

Leave the doll with the person if they engage positively with it.

If the person begins to lose interest in the doll or it is ignored, remove the doll, thanking the person for joining you in that moment.

As with all activities, it is essential that you have a good biography of the person before you engage in working with the doll. A doll can be a highly emotive symbol of love or pain, of parenthood or the yearning for parenthood, for success or loss.

You will know from the person's biography what response *may* be elicited when working with the doll; however, do not make assumptions about gender and do not assume that someone who enjoyed dolls many years ago will do so now. Do not exclude an individual from a potentially positive experience in the assumption that the person did not like dolls in the past.

Be mindful of your own attitudes and feelings about dolls and the therapeutic use of dolls. This is an opportunity to be truly person-centred and to possibly enter a humbling, enriched world.

FOOT SPA

Foot spas are available from a variety of sources including chemists and supermarkets. They will come with comprehensive instructions which you must follow *at all times*.

The foot spa can be used with people at all levels and is particularly beneficial for individuals at *sensory* and *reflex* activity levels of ability.

It is important to follow the preparation guidelines as it can take a short while to set up the foot spa – you do not want to lose an opportunity to engage a person in this activity by losing their attention early on.

As with all the activities, it is important that you know the person well. You need to consider how the person responds to touch, whether they like water, how they respond to noise and vibration, and whether they like their feet being touched.

You might want to consider introducing the use of the foot spa as part of an individual's self-care routine. It is important that you introduce this activity slowly and with sensitivity.

Ensure that the person is seated in an upright chair to maintain good posture and optimum positioning to enable them to engage fully. The person may like to have someone sitting alongside them for reassurance and affirmation.

Remove the person's shoes and socks/stockings/tights. Reinforce this by explaining to the person what you are doing. (They may not understand your words but will appreciate your reassuring, calm tone.)

Gently rub or stroke the person's feet for a few moments to enable them to begin to identify with the sensory stimulus and assist with orientation to that part of the body.

Introduce the foot spa slowly. Perhaps you could drip a little water over the person's feet to enable them to experience a changed sensation. Carefully monitor the person's response. If they show negative response signs such as grimacing or crying out, withdrawing the foot, or a change in posture, end the activity immediately and offer reassurance. If the person remains calm, shows positive signs, smiles, laughs, offers attention, then continue.

Gently place the person's feet – one at a time – into the foot spa. Again, continually monitor the person's response. Gently massage the feet in the water, allowing the water to gently splash. Use verbal and non-verbal communication throughout: eye contact, smiling, saying 'oooh', 'aaah' and 'how nice'. Continue to monitor the response, and if the person appears to be enjoying the sensation, consider changing the setting of the foot spa to whirl and heat or massage only, or whirl, heat and massage.

Remember that too much sensory stimulus can cause distress, so carefully monitor the response at each stage.

You may wish to use the relaxation music in this pack as gentle background music while the person enjoys the activity. Check the temperature of the water at all times, and do not allow it to become too hot or too cold. Monitor the response of the person and agree when the activity is complete.

Carefully lift the feet – one at a time – out of the foot spa and remove them to a safe distance. Gently towel dry the person's feet, again monitoring their response and reinforcing your actions with verbal and non-verbal communication.

Apply talcum powder or moisturizer if required. Replace socks/tights/stockings and shoes.

Sit quietly with the person for a few moments, talk about the activity and thank them for joining in.

COLOURED LIGHT SPHERE

A coloured light sphere can be used with people at the *sensory* and *reflex* activity levels of ability.

The use of slow-moving light can be used to rehabilitate some of the visual skills of a person with cognitive impairment. When used therapeutically, with another person's facilitation, the lamp can help the person to focus attention on, and to track the movement of, the multi-coloured light rays.

Use of the coloured light sphere can also help to reduce stress-related behaviour. You may wish to use the relaxation music playlist in this pack as gentle background music while the person enjoys the activity.

Introduce the person to the coloured light sphere while it is switched off. Describe what it will do: 'This ball will give off lots of different coloured lights'; and ask if the person would like to see it: 'Would you like to see?' Explain that you are going to switch it on and when the rays begin to move use your verbal and non-verbal communication skills to facilitate the person to see them: 'Look', 'Watch', 'See the red one'. Use the person's name also to stimulate their attention to your communication and use pointing to help direct their gaze.

Carefully monitor the person's response to the moving light rays. If they show negative response signs, which may include withdrawal, rocking, tense posture or crying out, end the activity immediately and offer reassurance.

If the person remains calm, shows positive signs, smiles, laughs, offers attention, then continue. You may find it helpful, once the person's attention has been captured, to remain silent and enable the person to enjoy the experience.

Monitoring the response of the person, agree when the activity is complete. Switch off the coloured light sphere and sit quietly with the person for a few moments, talk about the activity and thank them for joining in.

VIBRATING PILLOW

Vibrating pillows are available from some of the sources listed at the start of this chapter. They will come with comprehensive instructions which you must follow *at all times*. The vibrating pillow can be used with people at the *sensory* and *reflex* activity levels of ability.

Users at a *sensory* activity level will be able to activate the vibrations and turn them off themselves. This can give them a sense of control over their own environment and a sense of achievement in making something happen. The vibrating pillow is also useful for people functioning at a *reflex* activity level who may have difficulty initiating any movement of their own and rely on direct stimulation of the senses in order to make a movement in response.

The sensation of vibration can offer powerful stimulation as well as a means of keeping the person's attention and calming troubled behaviour. The vibrating pillow is made from a tactile fabric which the person can be encouraged to stroke and smooth as an introduction to this activity.

Explain to the person that this pillow can vibrate and show them what happens when you apply pressure to start the vibrations and release pressure for the vibrations to stop. Use your own body language, smiling and nodding, to give the message that this is acceptable and enjoyable, and use spoken language: 'ooh', 'aah', 'lovely'.

Encourage the person at a *sensory* activity level to apply pressure and to release it themselves and acknowledge when they have achieved it: 'Well done, it's working', 'Good for you, it's switched off'. Encourage the person to experiment with experiencing the vibrations through the hands, back, stomach, feet.

Assist the person at a *reflex* activity level to apply pressure, or place it in a position where pressure is naturally applied – behind the small of the back or under the feet.

Carefully monitor the person's response to the vibrations. If they show negative response signs, which may include withdrawal, rocking, tense posture or crying out, end the activity immediately and offer reassurance.

If the person remains calm, shows positive signs, smiles, laughs, offers attention, then continue. You may find it helpful, once the person's attention has been captured, to remain silent and enable the person to enjoy the experience.

Monitoring the response of the person, agree when the activity is complete. Remove the vibrating pillow and sit quietly with the person for a few moments, talk about the activity and thank them for joining in.

The person must not be left unaccompanied with this vibrating pillow, as prolonged sensory stimulation may be uncomfortable and distressing.

BUMPIE BALL

The 'interestingly' named bumpie ball can be used with people at both *sensory* and *reflex* activity levels. The texture, colour, shape of the ball can be extremely attractive and a little intriguing.

People at the *sensory* activity level will be able to grasp the ball and can be encouraged to explore its facets. People at a *reflex* activity level can be stimulated by the ball when used as a massager.

Offer the ball to the person who is at the *sensory* activity level. You may present it as an 'interesting object' which you would like to share and explore with the person. Allow the person to take the ball and wait a few moments to see how they respond. If the person's attention is drawn to the ball, they look at it or perhaps move it around on their hand, reinforce this response with positive comments, for example 'it feels nice', 'it's soft', 'what a lovely colour'.

Encourage the person to sense the ball through sight and touch. Allow the person to explore the ball with both hands. They may pick at the bumps on the ball or stroke it. Accompany this with calm, reassuring comments, constantly monitoring the person's response. The person may take the ball to their mouth. (You can wash the ball after it has been used.)

The person may throw the ball towards you or pass it back to you. Facilitate this opportunity for turn taking and promoting a sense of agency by returning the ball to the person, either a gentle throw or placing the ball in the person's hands or lap. Maintain eye contact with the person, smile and mirror their positive responses.

It may be possible to engage with more than one person, by passing or throwing the ball to others in combination with saying their name. It is *vital* that you ensure that you have gained the attention of the person before throwing or even passing the ball to them. The person must be prepared to receive the ball otherwise they will be startled and distressed.

Constantly monitor the response of the person. The person may throw the ball away, be unresponsive or uninterested in the ball, allowing it to sit in their lap without touching it. In this instance, remove the ball and consider offering a different type of stimulus according to the person's preference.

If the person does show interest in the ball and appears stimulated by it, you may consider including the ball in a 'feely bag' containing other objects such as a silk scarf, fur, cotton wool or a necklace of beads which you can take out in turn for the person to touch and explore. The person might enjoy watching you blow the ball up, engaging with their sense of hearing – and fun!

For a person at the *reflex* activity level, the bumpie ball can be used as a massager. Ensure that you have gained the attention of the person, seek eye contact or movement towards you in recognition of your voice, or touch their hand or shoulder. The person should be seated in an upright chair and in a good position. Place the ball in the person's lap and lift one of their hands on top of it. Constantly monitor the response of the person. If they cry out or withdraw their hand, remove the ball immediately and give reassurance.

By studying the person's positive non-verbal responses, continue with the activity by placing your hand over their hand and gently moving the ball in rhythmic patterns.

If the person is willing and responds positively, take the ball from under the person's hand and gently roll it up their arm. Continuously monitor the response of the person as you roll the ball up the arm and across the back of their shoulders and gently down the other arm. It is hoped that the sensation of pressure will be stimulating for the person or an enjoyable, relaxing experience. (It will be helpful to have a colleague with you so that they can monitor the person's response as you roll the ball across their shoulders.)

You may wish to use the relaxation music playlist included in this pack to reinforce the gentle, relaxing atmosphere.

Again, your knowledge of the person and constant monitoring of their responses will guide you as to whether to place the ball under the person's feet. Sit at the person's feet ensuring that you have gained their attention. Gently remove the shoe from one of the feet and massage the foot to enable the person to recognize the stimulation to that part of their body. Lift the foot and place it on top of the ball. Holding gently to the foot and lower limb, allow the limb to move rhythmically as the ball sways and moves beneath. Repeat with the other foot, constantly monitoring the person's response.

If the person cries out, withdraws the limb or expresses ill-being, remove the ball immediately, allowing the foot to rest gently back into position, and offer reassurance.

Monitoring the response of the person, agree when the activity has ended. Replace the person's shoes and perhaps sit quietly with them or listen to the relaxation music playlist.

Thank the person for joining in the activity with you and ensure that the person is aware that the activity has ended.

LAVENDER MOISTURIZING BODY LOTION

We interact with the environment and people around us through stimulation of our senses. When people are asked 'Which of the senses would you least like to lose?' they often have difficulty in deciding. It is difficult to imagine such a loss and the impact this would have on our life and abilities.

In working with people with cognitive impairments we have the opportunity of engaging and communicating in a variety of ways, not least through the sense of smell.

It must be remembered that not everyone has the same experience of smell, and that this sense may be damaged through neurological impairment or the normal ageing process. Some people may never have had a sense of smell, and for some this may have been heightened.

In terms of orientation, smell is invaluable. For many, the smell of pine, cinnamon and spiced fruit will make them think of Christmas. Who can smell freshly-cut grass or a sea breeze without thinking of summer?

Memory and the sense of smell are both associated with the function of the temporal lobe in the brain. It is not surprising that there is such a close relationship. Lavender has long been considered one of the most recognizable of smells. It has associations with clean, crisp linen, lavender bags, perfume and even sweets. Many people have grown lavender in their garden and immediately recognize its aroma. Latterly, the benefits of lavender as an essential oil have been recognized in terms of relaxation and healing. While essential oils can be contra-indicated for some people and should only be used by qualified aromatherapists, it is possible to gain some benefits from moisturizers and lotions that contain these oils. Lavender moisturizing body lotion recommended for this pack can be used with people at both *sensory* and *reflex* activity levels.

As with all activities, it is essential to know the person's history, likes and dislikes and, in this instance, whether they have a sense of smell! (If they don't have a sense of smell, you would adapt the activity accordingly.)

For a person at the *sensory* activity level the body lotion can be used in a variety of ways, depending on the person's response.

Show the person the body lotion bottle informing them that there is lavender-scented lotion in it. This may elicit an immediate response. The person may take the bottle from you. If the person would like to remove the lid themselves, encourage them to do so or offer the necessary support to assist them.

Encourage the person to smell the lotion in the bottle. Make sure that they do not breathe in too deeply or frequently as this may cause them to feel dizzy or hyperventilate. You smell it too.

Encourage communication: 'What a lovely smell!', 'What does that remind you of?', 'Mmm, how lovely', 'Do you like it?' Use non-verbal communication too: smiling, closing eyes and exaggerating inhalation or maintaining eye contact. The person may be able to spontaneously reminisce; encourage this with open questions and reflection.

Of course, the person may not be able to smell it, so do not labour the above. The person also may not like the smell or it may hold negative associations – be prepared for this.

Ask if the person would like to have some lotion placed on a hand. If so, ensure that the person's clothing is protected by rolling up sleeves and placing a towel over the lap. The person may pour lotion into their hands spontaneously and begin to massage them. Again, reinforce this with positive communication, talking about how it feels, reinforcing reminiscence, recognizing that the smell may become more pungent.

If the person does not put lotion onto their hands independently, ask if you can do this for them and constantly monitor the person's response. Be aware of the temperature of the lotion as it may be quite cold when coming directly from the bottle.

In both cases, constantly monitor the person's response. Ask if the person would like you to give them a hand massage. If they agree, the following massage guide may be useful:

- Ensure that you have adequate moisturizing lotion on your hands. Carefully rub your hands together to warm the lotion.
- Take the person's hand in yours, and holding it palm down use your thumbs to gently massage the back of the hand.
- Turn the hand over and gently massage the palm with your thumbs.
- Palm to palm, use circular movements over the person's hand and fingers.
- Massage each digit in turn, starting with the thumb and continuing, finishing with the little finger.
- Use stroking movements over the palm and back of the hand, extending up over the wrist to midway between wrist and elbow.
- Circle the hand and wrist with your hands using rhythmical, gentle upward and downward, flowing movements as your hands overlap.
- Use downward stroking movements over the back and palm of the person's hand.
- Once the massage is complete, use a towel to remove any excess lotion.

Thank the person for participating in the activity with you and ask them how they feel. Sit quietly with them before formally ending the activity.

You could use the body lotion as a resource for a small group of people, all at the *sensory* activity level, by developing an 'olfactory stimulation kit' or 'smelly box'.

Transfer items such as the body lotion, coffee essence, washing powder, mint mouthwash, marmite, brandy, herbs or vinegar into lidded containers.

Present the activity as a 'smell quiz', allowing participants to smell each item in turn and see if they can identify it and reminisce about it.

For people at the *reflex* activity level, you can use the body lotion in the same way as for the hand massage activity. Make sure that you continuously monitor the response of the individual and adjust the activity accordingly.

You may also wish to use the body lotion in conjunction with the foot spa included in this pack.

Play the relaxation music to accompany the massage if appropriate, but be careful not to offer too much sensory stimulation as this can be distressing for the individual.

Ensure that participants do not attempt to ingest the contents of the containers and do not hyperventilate.

SUMMARY

Part 2 of this book has provided you with ideas that can be facilitated to support people at different PAL levels of ability to engage in activities with meaning and enjoyment. It is not, of course, an exhaustive list but is intended to illustrate how, with imagination, enthusiasm and skill, it is possible to present the world to the person so that they can enjoy a high-quality lifestyle. By doing so, you will not only elevate the well-being of those you care for but you will also find true satisfaction in knowing that you have made a real and positive difference to the person's experience of living with dementia. Completing the PAL Engagement Measure for individuals as they engage with you in the same activity over a period of time will support you to measure and evidence this impact and provide a source of pride to you and the organization that you work with.